HOME SPA

HOME
SPA

ANNE HARDING
with JANICE BIEHN

KEY PORTER BOOKS

National Library of Canada Cataloguing in Publication Data

Harding, Anne
     Home spa / Anne Harding ; with Janice Biehn.

ISBN 1-55263-635-6 (bound).—ISBN 1-55013-694-1 (pbk.)

     1. Health. 2. Skin—Care and hygiene. I. Biehn, Janice II. Title.

RA776.H365 1997	613	C95-931629-9

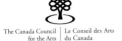

The Canada Council | Le Conseil des Arts
for the Arts | du Canada

ONTARIO ARTS COUNCIL
CONSEIL DES ARTS DE L'ONTARIO

The publisher gratefully acknowledges the support of the Canada Council for the Arts and the Ontario Arts Council for its publishing program. We acknowledge the support of the Government of Ontario through the Ontario Media Development Corporation's Ontario Book Initiative.

We acknowledge the financial support of the Government of Canada through the Book Publishing Industry Development Program (BPIDP) for our publishing activities.

Key Porter Books Limited
70 The Esplanade
Toronto, Ontario
Canada M5E 1R2

www.keyporter.com

Illustrations: John Lightfoot
Design: Jean Lightfoot Peters
Electronic formatting: Heidi Palfrey

Printed and bound in Canada

04 05 06 07 08 5 4 3 2 1

Contents

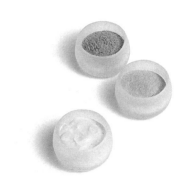

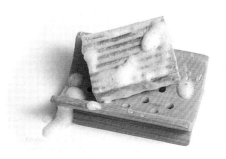

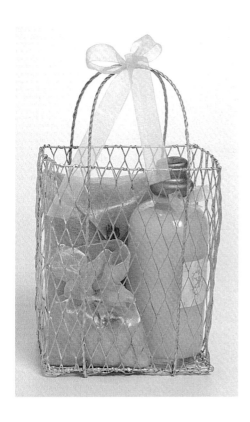

Body and Beauty Treatments 75

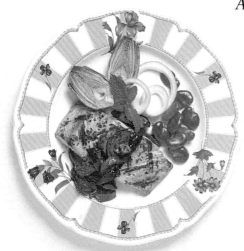

The Home Spa 97

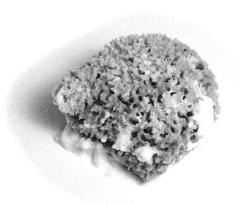

Where to Find It 110

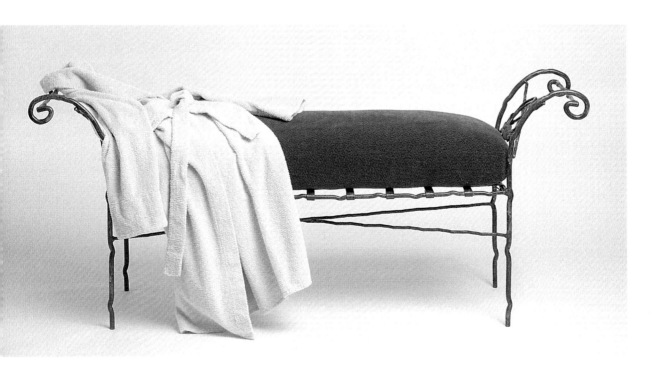

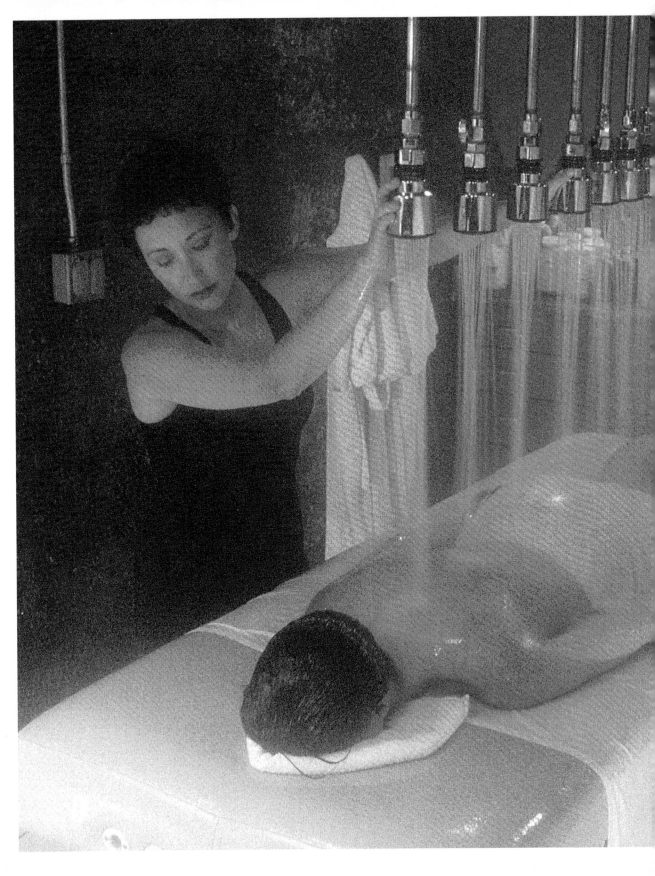

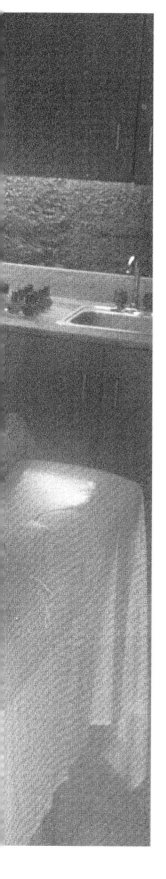

Introduction

It's hard to imagine what soaking in a tub of mud feels like until you've done it yourself. The dense, pudding-like muck simultaneously keeps you afloat and weighs you down. With your head leaning back against an inflatable pillow, a diligent attendant carefully wiping your perspiring brow, you begin to feel weightless. The scent of jasmine wafts through the steamy, tiled room; new-age music flows around you. The centuries-old mud supposedly draws toxins from your body. But even if you're skeptical about mud's curative powers, you can't deny how the experience makes you feel—relaxed.

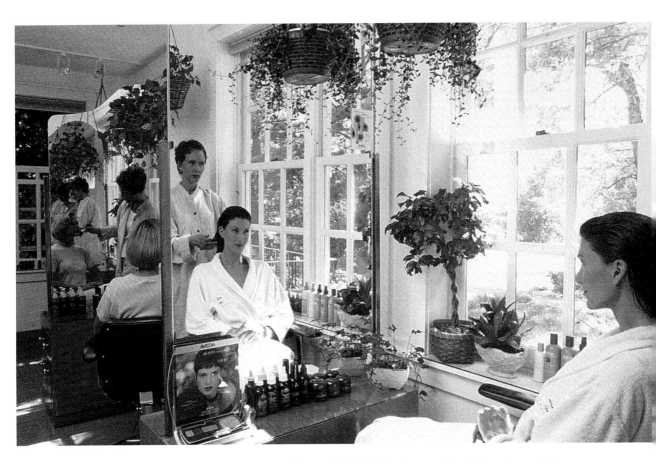

Spa boutiques give you the option of relaxing in the middle of a hectic work day.

After you've had 10 minutes of squishing the mud between your toes, the attendant helps you out of the tub and sprays you clean. Take a sip of cool water enhanced with lemon and cucumber slices. Then don your fluffy white robe and float to the next treatment room for a Sea Salt Glow. First the attendant stimulates and massages your skin with a high-power hose. Then, on a massage table, she rubs a salty paste into your skin to exfoliate dead skin cells. Most of the salt comes off with a gentle scrub; any remaining grains are sure to be blasted off while you're lying under the bank of eight shower nozzles, each gently pulsating and massaging a different section of your body.

Pat yourself dry and return to the massage table, which is now draped in warm flannel sheets, one to lie on and one to keep you warm.

Imagine how much less stressful your day would be if you and everyone you interact with started the day like this. It's an elaborate way to bathe, but the pampering of a spa experience is well worth it.

For centuries, the word *spa* has referred to a place where natural curative springs flow. Bath, England, and Baden-Baden, Germany, are two of the most famous examples of spas. But over the years, *spa* has evolved to include body massages, steam baths, saunas and all manner of aesthetic beautifiers such as manicures, pedicures and facials. In the late 1970s, savvy salon operators recognized that not everyone had the time or money to get away for a spa vacation, so spa boutiques began cropping up in major cities across the continent. In the midst of the hustle and bustle of urban chaos, these white-tiled oases have helped millions get the spa break they need.

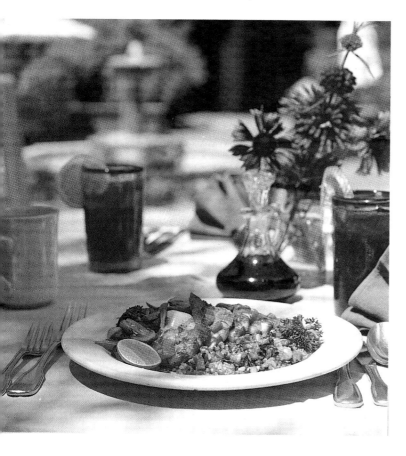

Heart-friendly, fat-free dishes like this characterize spa cuisine.

A long soak in a warm tub rejuvenates the body and the soul.

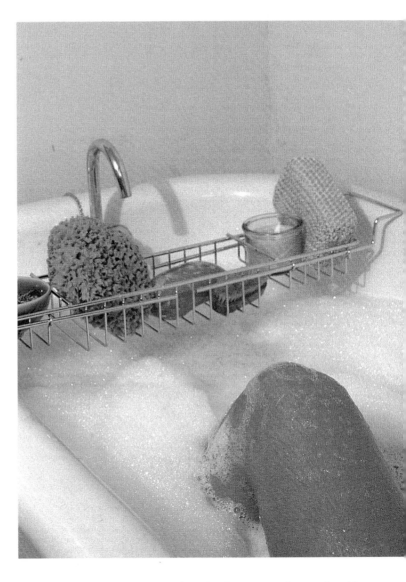

Most recently, the notion of spa has become such a marketable one that cosmetic companies have raced to add the three-letter word to packages of toners, moisturizers and body scrubs. Then there's spa cuisine—the latest in a long line of culinary styles to crop up in the 1980s and 1990s—characterized by low-fat, heart-friendly dishes served up in healthful portions.

In our quest to defy aging and keep harmful stress at bay, *spa* has come to be associated with all things healthy. It suggests a lifestyle that includes physical fitness, emotional fitness, good nutrition and skin care, and recognizes that all these facets of our health are inextricably linked. When we neglect one element, one or more of the others slumps. Indulge in one too many candy bars? Watch your skin take the brunt. No time to take that morning walk? Watch your temper shorten. And of course, if stress starts weighing you down, watch your whole body fall apart.

A week at a spa, or even a few days for that matter, helps you integrate fitness, nutrition and relaxation for a healthier, happier you. The good news is that you don't have to go to a secluded spa or even a downtown salon to destress.

- We'll teach you how to live the spa life every day. Give stress the boot with some simple relaxation techniques and dietary strategies.
- Follow our 10 easy steps to better health—lifestyle changes that you can adopt at your own pace without starving yourself. Learn how to increase your stamina by boosting your metabolism, and how to eat healthy meals in restaurants. Get hooked on exercise without "making it burn" for a change.
- With stress control, good nutrition and an exercise strategy in the bag, you're ready for a little spa pampering. Turn a ho-hum bath into an aromatherapy treatment. Soothe your aching muscles with a reflexology massage, or try a homemade mask to give your skin a refreshing lift. We've organized the day for you. Now it's up to you to make the time to do it.

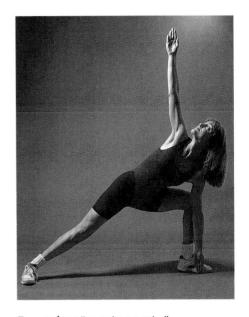

Forget about "no pain, no gain." Exercise is easy.

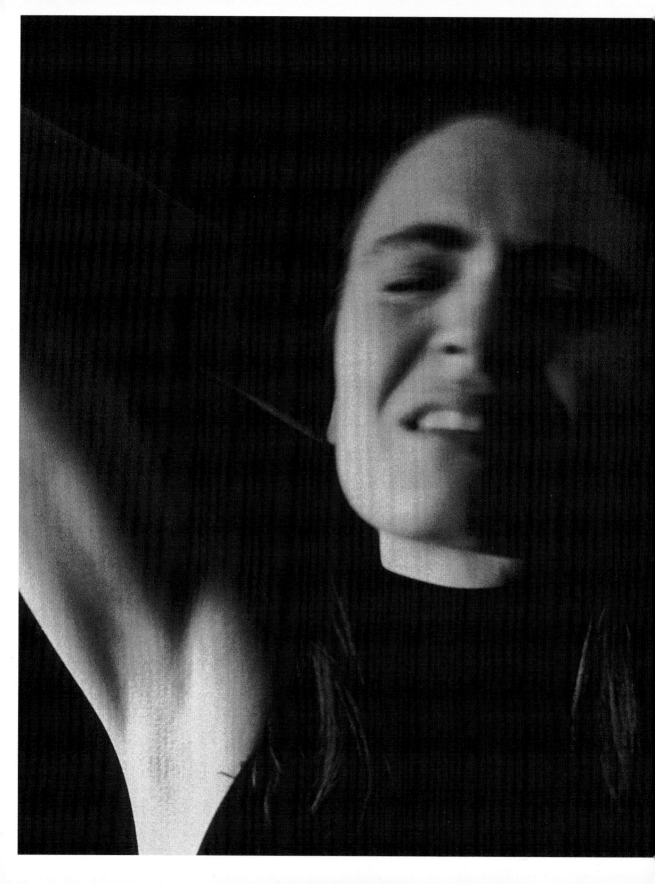

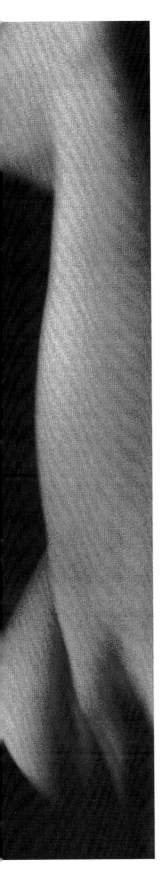

A Few Words about Stress

Skeptics about adopting a spa lifestyle might say the point of a spa is to get away—get away from the house, the kids, the dog, work. But let's face it, practicality and money often stand in the way. The truth is, *spa* is more a state of mind than an actual place. The first key to unlocking the door is to learn to recognize stress, in some cases live with it, but in most cases, eradicate it.

We all experience a certain amount of stress in our lives. Imagine Michelangelo hanging from the rafters of the Sistine Chapel, or the settlers of this continent forging their way across rugged terrain without the benefit of sport utility vehicles. Today's stresses seem almost petty by comparison, but our bodies still undergo the same biological reaction. We struggle with our finances, fight traffic, battle disease, defy age: it's no wonder life seems too hard some days.

Learning to deal with stress is one of the most important ways to prevent illness. Too much stress can interfere with basic bodily functions—causing anything from nausea to diarrhea to insomnia. Inability to handle stress can lead to alcoholism, smoking and drug abuse. It can also aggravate heart disease, cancer, diabetes, asthma, irritable bowel syndrome, tuberculosis, multiple sclerosis and rheumatoid arthritis.

So what is stress? It's a stimulus that elicits a genetically programmed reaction in any living creature—the one-celled amoeba, a dandelion, a dog or its owner. In the animal kingdom, the instinct to protect ourselves is strong. In primitive man, for example, stress reactions helped preserve and propagate the species. When the caveman was under attack, his breathing accelerated, his heart rate shot up. The blood flow to the muscles increased, and his body was deriving peak energy levels from carbohydrate and fat deposits. His blood developed a greater tendency to clot. These biological stress reactions were practical to anyone encountering the occasional wooly mammoth.

Today, of course, our need to call on these automatic defense mechanisms is far less. But the instant you have to step on the brakes to avoid hitting a small child playing in the street, your body's stress reactions kick in. You have to pull over briefly to gather yourself after that moment of panic. That surge of adrenalin usually requires a few minutes to subside.

Is that a familiar feeling? If your stress buttons are being pushed way too often, your body may react in a number of ways. Know the common physical and psychological symptoms of excess stress so you can begin to make changes to avoid it.

• Frequent headaches or dizziness

- Low-grade infections (fevers)
- Increase or decrease of appetite
- Excessive smoking, drinking or use of tranquilizers
- Muscular aches and pains
- Nervous tics
- Insomnia, excessive sleeping or nightmares
- Acne or rashes
- Crying easily or feeling that you might
- Constipation or diarrhea
- Chest pain or shortness of breath
- Frigidity or impotence, and loss of interest in sex
- High blood pressure
- Excessive sweating when not exercising
- Stuttering
- Nausea, vomiting or stomach pain
- Grinding of teeth
- Lethargy or excessive fatigue
- Inability to concentrate
- Rapid or hard heart beating when not exercising
- Irritability, impatience, bad temper
- Cold, clammy, clenched hands or loss of feeling in hands
- Sudden burst of energy followed by lethargy
- Finger tapping, foot tapping, pencil tapping
- Depression, anxiety, fear or panic attacks
- Hives or blotches
- Excessive coughing
- Excessive unusual hair loss
- Hyperactivity, restlessness or jumpiness
- Dry mouth or throat
- Biting lips or fingernails
- Frequent colds, flu or other infections
- Oversensitivity, emotional and/or physical

If you're experiencing one or more of these symptoms, it could be stress-related. Your body may be sending up flares that you are not doing all you could to stay healthy. Maybe it's time to examine your current lifestyle. See your doctor to rule out any other causes.

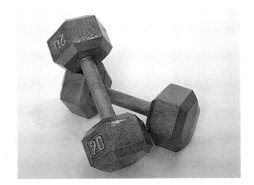

Physical fitness is crucial to keeping harmful stress at bay.

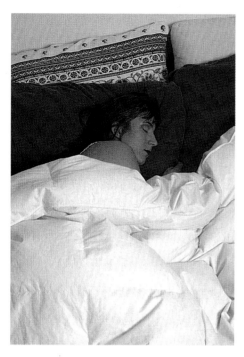

Lack of sleep could be contributing to a stressful state of mind.

Taking Care of Stress

Many experts recommend the following basic concepts for managing stress:

- Learn a relaxation technique appropriate for you.
- Think about making changes in your life to reduce stress, but don't make too many in a short period of time.
- Exercise—it releases tensions and benefits health.
- Eat well—stress robs your body of nutrients, making you more vulnerable to illness.
- Take time off.
- Decrease the noise and confusion around you.
- Talk to friends, relatives or professionals about your problems. Don't hold it all in.
- Join support groups that include people who are in the same situation as you.
- Get regular physical checkups.
- Plan your work, manage your time. Set realistic goals.
- Avoid unnecessary stress when you have a choice.
- Get enough sleep.
- Realize that it may be necessary to quit a job or change a situation in order to be happier.
- Get involved in hobbies, interests and other people.
- Recognize what you can and what you cannot change. For those things that are beyond your control, accept them.
- Take breaks in your daily routine to pamper yourself. Have fun.

Five Exercises for Destressing

In some ways, stress can be a state of mind. What one person finds exciting may leave another frightened. Most people thrive on a certain amount of stress—finding your ideal level is a process of trial and error. Balancing the optimum level of stress with periods of relaxation is the key to making stress work for you. But most of us can't, or don't know how to, relax. The following exercises are designed to help change a stressful state of mind into a calm, peaceful one.

Meditate You don't have to practice the lotus position and listen to sitar music to enjoy the benefits of meditation. It's a technique to help you clear your mind and give it a break. Meditation is most successful when done in a comfortable, private place without distractions—in a warm tub, for example, or even your parked car after the drive home.

Start by closing your eyes and focusing on one peaceful word or image. Many meditation instructors suggest picturing a sunny beach with the ocean waves lapping at your toes. When your boss or bank manager enters your mind, send them packing and return to the warm sand. You're erasing your mind's slate of shoulds, coulds, dos and don'ts and allowing yourself the luxury of a peaceful break. The mere act of taking five minutes for yourself, regardless of how successful the meditation exercise, is an important first step in reducing stress.

Some meditation instructors also incorporate chanting into their routines. Take a deep cleansing breath. When exhaling, let the breath make a sound. Gradually change the huffing and puffing to a deep guttural "Ooooohm" and feel the tension leave your body. You may

HAVE A KAVA KAVA

There are several herbal remedies for stress caused by anxiety, insomnia and muscle aches, for example (see the section on aromatherapy on p. 90), but the number one stress kicker is the South American herbal staple called kava kava. This member of the pepper family does everything from relaxing muscles and enhancing moods to promoting alertness.

You can take kava kava in capsule form three times a day, or in juice or tea (extract in water). Within a few hours, or possibly a few days, the relaxing effects should begin to wash over you.

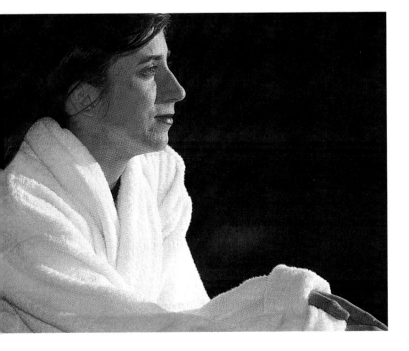

Learn to destress with a daily five-minute daydream break.

YOU ARE WHAT YOU EAT

Can diet affect stress? Definitely. Stress is our bodies' reaction to change. Every time we experience a new situation our bodies produce more adrenalin, which gives us extra energy to deal with the challenge at hand, be it the excitement of a new job or the frustration of a crying baby. This energy is fueled by the nutrients we store from the foods we eat. Too much stress can drain our supplies of these nutrients, leaving us with little or no fuel for our daily energy needs. This can result in weakness, fatigue and—yes—more stress. The key to eating for less stress is to avoid foods that aggravate our stress response, and to increase our bodies' stores of the nutrients we need to handle stressful situations.

Limit caffeine and alcohol Like adrenalin, caffeine is a stimulant. Too much caffeine can imitate that adrenalin surge, or if you are already under stress, it's like a double dose. Caffeine is found in coffee, tea, chocolate and many soft drinks, especially colas. Limit caffeine in general; avoid it if you're already under stress.

Alcohol, on the other hand, is a depressant. While a stiff martini at the end of a tough day may bring short-term relief of stress, more than one can become habit-forming. And it's a Band-Aid cure, masking the actual cause of the stress in exchange for immediate gratification.

Eat Vitamin C rich foods Your adrenal glands, which produce adrenalin, use Vitamin C during episodes of physical stress. Illness or injury can deplete Vitamin C. Eating a variety of fresh fruits and vegetables—especially citrus fruits—can help ensure that your body has adequate Vitamin C. You can also check with your doctor or a nutritionist about a Vitamin C supplement.

Eat protein and complex carbohydrates Your body also uses more protein and complex carbohydrates when you're under stress. Good sources of protein include peas, beans, fish, poultry and lean red meats. Complex carbohydrates are found in fruits, vegetables and whole-grain products such as breads, cereals and pasta. Avoid refined flours and sugars as these can compound stress responses.

feel a little self-conscious at first, but once you get the hang of it, the outside world doesn't matter.

Daydream The teacher may look reproachfully at the student who gazes dreamily out the window, but make no mistake, that day-dreaming kid is the happier, healthier one. Daydreaming, or visualization, encourages that same feeling of tranquility, but instead of focusing on just one single peaceful thought, you think about an entire relaxing environment in full detail.

Take the meditation image, for example: you're lying on a beach in Fiji, water whooshing gently on the shore. In a daydream, you take the image a step further. Imagine a waiter bringing you a frothy, fruity drink. Perhaps you get up for a little swim. You lazily roll over and someone magically rubs suntan lotion on your back.

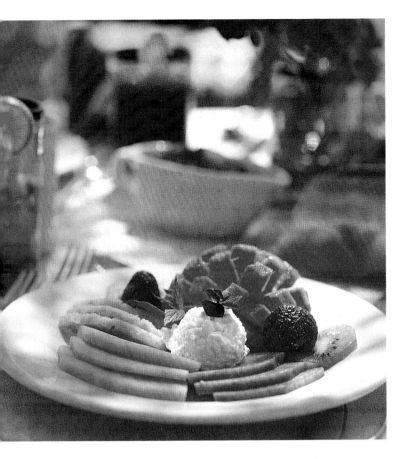

A balanced diet helps keep stress in check.

Daydreaming has one advantage over meditation. Generally, you can keep your eyes open. One woman we know "saves up" her daydreams to make slow-moving commutes more pleasurable.

Deep Muscle Relaxation Muscle tension is one of the most common reactions to stress. Deep muscle relaxation helps you push the stress from your body by tensing and relaxing various muscle groups. The whole process takes about 15 minutes and can be done almost anywhere. First, sit (or lie) down and close your eyes. Tense your facial muscles (purse your lips, squeeze your forehead, etc.); hold for five seconds, then relax. Now move on to the neck and shoulders—tense, hold, relax. Continue doing this with your arms, hands, back, abdominals, hips, legs and feet. By the time you're done, your muscle tension will have drained away and you'll feel revived and refreshed.

Spa treatments are therapy for the body and the mind.

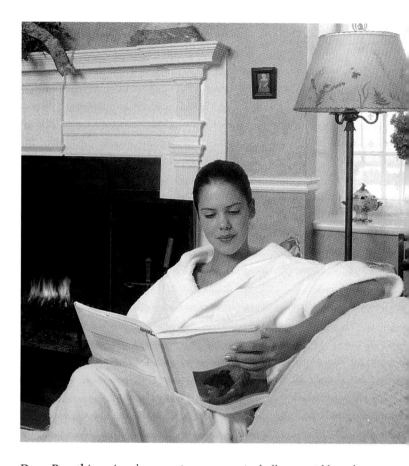

Deep Breathing Another reaction to stress is shallow, rapid breathing. Deep, slow breathing can interrupt your stress response and help you relax. First, clear the "stale" air from your lungs by exhaling slowly through your mouth until your lungs feel completely empty. Then, inhale through your nose until you begin to feel your abdomen rise. Hold for five seconds, then exhale and begin the cycle again. Repeat this exercise four to five times whenever you feel tense. Deep, abdominal breathing takes only a few seconds and can be done anywhere. So, when you find yourself tense and irritable, stop and take a breather.

The Power of Suggestion Autogenic or self-regulating suggestion proves stress-busting is mind over matter. When stress overtakes you, sit down and close your eyes. Suggest a calming mental notion to yourself, such as "My arms are as light as feathers, I am calm and peaceful," and so on. You can focus on all parts of your body that feel tense. By putting your mind to it, you can talk yourself into a more relaxed, tranquil frame of mind.

The Pamper Principle

Spa treatments have a twofold effect on stress: physically, you're afforded a chance to rest and rejuvenate. Most treatments, such as a massage or a steam bath, for example, also give your circulatory system a boost. Psychologically, the effect of a spa treatment is even more pronounced. Not only do you give your brain a break, but you're also telling yourself that you deserve a break. Nothing can be more enlightening or more soul-satisfying.

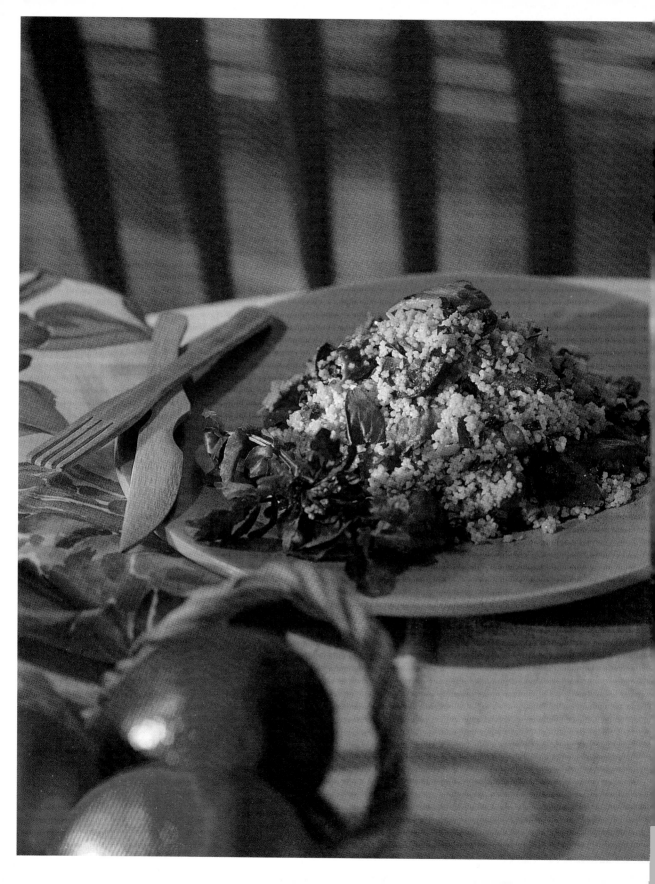

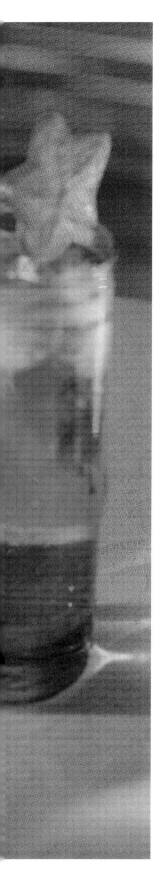

10 Easy Steps to Better Health

Gone are the days of "fat farms" where clients starved themselves and wrapped their bodies in cellophane while running 10 miles. Most of today's spa resorts (with the exception of some specialty retreats) have ditched the old "no pain, no gain" adage. Spas recognize that combining low-fat, gourmet dishes with a reasonable and relaxing exercise program is the best way to maintain a comfortable weight and improve overall health.

The Exercise-Nutrition Connection

Food energy, measured in calories, comes in three forms: carbohydrates, protein and fats. The other nutrients, including vitamins, minerals and water, help your body use the food energy as well as perform other basic bodily functions.

Metabolism alone uses up a significant amount of calories every day. All physical activity requires more calories, and exercise uses still more. The more you exercise, the more energy you use. When more energy is taken in than is used up, the excess energy is stored as body fat. There are 3,500 calories of food energy in a pound of fat. So, to lose a pound of fat, you must create a deficit of 3,500 calories by decreasing what you take in and/or increasing what you expend.

Far too many people try to lose weight by only restricting food. This is an ineffective and dangerous way to attempt weight loss, resulting in loss of muscle as well as fat. It can also cause metabolism to slow down, which means even fewer calories are being used for energy and more are being stored as fat. The best way to lose body fat is to eat moderately less food from a balanced diet and to increase exercise—especially of the aerobic type. This will result in a quicker and safer loss of body fat, preserve muscle tissue and increase metabolism.

Most of today's spas offer an in-depth lifestyle assessment based on eating patterns, food choices and level of fitness. Nutritionists and fitness experts provide strategies on how to manage your weight and get worked up about working out. In our 10 steps, we hope to give you the same tools to examine your own lifestyle and evaluate where you can make your own changes.

1 Down with Fat, Up with Fiber

Ever since medical research linked high-fat foods with heart disease and some forms of cancer, fat has had a bad rap. Dietary fat (the fat we eat) produces fatty acids when digested. One such "essential" fatty acid—linoleic acid—helps us absorb fat-soluble vitamins.

There are three types of fat: saturated (bad), polyunsaturated (good) and monounsaturated, which is good if taken in moderation and not heated. Saturated fats are usually solid at room temperature and are found in animal fats—red meats, lard, poultry with skin and whole milk dairy products, including butter. Palm and coconut oils are also highly saturated. These fats are known to contribute to higher levels of heart-damaging cholesterol, cardiovascular disease and many types of cancer. Unsaturated fats are found primarily in vegetable oils, such as safflower, sunflower and corn oils, that do not solidify at room temperature. Besides providing the body with linoleic acid, unsaturated fats have been shown to reduce cholesterol levels in some individuals, which in turn may reduce the risk of cardiovascular disease. Monounsaturated fats, found in olive, peanut and canola oils, are usually liquid at room temperature, but solid once refrigerated. No firm evidence has been provided linking monounsaturated fats with good health; however, cultures in which olive oil is a diet staple have shown lower rates of heart disease. Other recent studies have shown that when a monounsaturated oil replaces a saturated one, it may lower cholesterol.

While it's a good idea to watch your fat intake—even limit it to certain foods—you mustn't eliminate fat completely unless you're on a supervised diet. Daily fat consumption should not exceed 20% of your total calories. Of that 20%, no more than 10% should be from saturated fats. Most commercial calorie counters and food labels will list how many grams of fat are contained in specific food servings. (Multiply the number of grams of fat by 9—fat weighs nine calories per gram—to find out how many calories of fat a given serving contains.)

Before you start meticulously counting calories and counting every chocolate chip in that cookie, realize that it is healthy to have some body fat. Our bodies were programmed to store fat in case of emergency—kind of like a camel storing its water. Just how much fat we should carry around in our "humps" is the question.

$$\frac{\text{Lean body mass (bone and muscle density)}}{\text{Body fat (the visible, subcutaneous}} + \text{fat and the invisible intramuscular fat)}}{\text{Total body weight}}$$

When you gain fat, not only do you gain weight, you also displace the lean body mass, thus distorting the proportion of fat to lean body mass. In fact, when you step on that odious bathroom scale every morning, you are getting a deceptive reading about your body fat. And forget about that women's magazine mainstay of yore: ideal weight charts that basically took into account your height and age. It's ridiculous to suppose that all women who are 5'6" tall should weigh within the same 10-pound range. It's not your total weight that is important, but rather the proportion of body fat to lean body mass.

Experts have varying opinions about how much body fat is desirable. Generally, women are safe in the 18%-to-25% range; for men it's slightly lower at 15% to 20%.

How do you measure your body fat? The two accepted methods are skin-fold testing and hydrostatic weight. Calipers, which look like a giant set of pliers with a gauge in the middle, measure subcutaneous fat. A trained fitness consultant or nutritionist measures the thickness of fat under the skin by gently pinching it and pulling it away from the muscle. Hydrostatic, or underwater weighing, is considered to produce the most accurate measurement. In this method, you sit in a sling attached to a big scale submerged in a tank of water and release all the air from your system by exhaling deeply. The scale measures your lean body density. That figure, subtracted from your total body weight, equals your total body fat, which can be thus expressed as a percentage.

Unfortunately, these two methods aren't very convenient for most people, so you have to learn to recognize other markers. For example, your clothes are gradually becoming too tight, you get winded easily or high cholesterol runs in your family. Knowing you have too much body fat is usually obvious; finding ways to decrease body fat isn't.

Filling up on fiber is one way to fill the calorie gap and do your body good, too. Fiber, also known as roughage, comes from plant foods including fruits, vegetables and cereal grains. Regular doses of fiber in your diet can help prevent heart disease and cancer of the large bowel, breast and prostate, and also curb obesity by making you feel fuller, sooner. Soluble fibers, found in legumes, apples and some grains, such as oat bran, rye and barley, help lower cholesterol levels and stabilize blood sugar. Insoluble fibers, found in wheat bran and other cereals, promote regularity, thus keeping bowels healthier. Eating more soluble fibers without drinking more water can lead to constipation, so keep well hydrated. Lastly, fruits and vegetables contain a mixture of soluble and insoluble fibers.

Boost fiber by:

- eating an orange for breakfast, for example, instead of always drinking juice;
- sneaking a sprinkling of oat or wheat bran in ground beef when making burgers or meat loaf, or in breading for chicken or stuffing;
- keeping nuts on hand to add to salads or desserts.

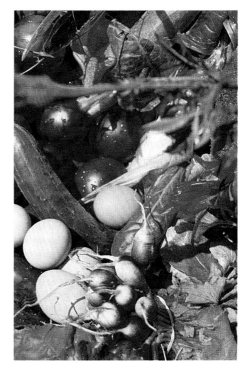

A high-fiber diet is rich in fruits and vegetables.

2 *Increase Your Fitness Level*

Cutting back on fat alone isn't going to change your percentage of body fat. To lose fat, you must change your body chemistry and increase its metabolism by exercising. If you already exercise, step up the pace. Exercising increases and tones muscle mass. It also burns calories, displacing fat with muscle.

This doesn't mean you're going to look like a muscle-bound body builder. Instead, you'll be operating at peak efficiency, with just enough fat to provide energy and to keep cells functioning properly.

Just 20 to 30 minutes of brisk walking three times a week, for example, is enough to improve heart and lung function. Longer periods will burn calories, especially fat calories. Contrary to the image that was popularized in the early 1980s by Jane Fonda and the like, aerobics doesn't necessarily mean squeezing into a Spandex outfit

MINERALS ESSENTIAL FOR HEALTH

Mineral	Major Body Functions	Results of Deficiency
Calcium	Bone and tooth formation, blood clotting, nerve transmission	Stunted growth, rickets, osteoporosis, convulsions
Chlorine	Formation of gastric juice, acid-base balance	Muscle cramps, mental apathy, reduced appetite
Fluorine	May be important in maintenance of bone structure	Higher frequency of tooth decay
Iron	Constituent of hemoglobin	Iron-deficiency anemia (weakness, reduced resistance)
Magnesium	Activates enzymes, involved in protein synthesis	Growth failure, behavioral disturbances, weakness, spasms
Phosphorus	Bone and tooth formation, acid-base balance	Weakness, demineralization of bone, loss of calcium
Potassium	Acid-base balance, body-water balance, nerve function	Muscular weakness, paralysis
Sodium	Acid-base balance, body-water balance, nerve function	Muscle cramps, mental apathy, reduced appetite
Sulfur	Constituent of active tissue compounds, cartilage and tendons	Related to intake and deficiency of sulfur amino acids
Zinc	Constituent of enzymes involved in digestion	Growth failure, lack of sexual maturation, loss of appetite, abnormal glucose tolerance

Results of Excess	Good Food Sources
Not reported in humans	Milk, cheese, dark green vegetables, dried legumes, sardines with bones, shellfish
Vomiting	Common table salt, seafood, milk, meat, eggs
Mottling of teeth, increased bone density, neurological disturbances	Drinking water, tea, coffee, seafood, rice, soybeans, spinach, gelatin, lettuce
Siderosis, cirrhosis of the liver	Liver, lean meats, legumes, whole grains, dark green vegetables, eggs, dark molasses, shrimp, oysters
Diarrhea	Whole grains, green leafy vegetables, nuts, meats, milk, legumes
Erosion of jaw	Milk, cheese, meat, fish, poultry, whole grains, legumes, nuts
Muscular weakness, death	Meat, milk, many fruits, legumes, vegetables
High blood pressure	Common table salt, seafood, milk, eggs, grains, most foods except fruit
Excess sulfur amino acids intake leads to poor growth	Protein foods (milk, cheese, meat, fish, poultry, eggs, legumes, nuts)
Fever, nausea, vomiting, diarrhea	Milk, liver, shellfish, herring, wheat bran

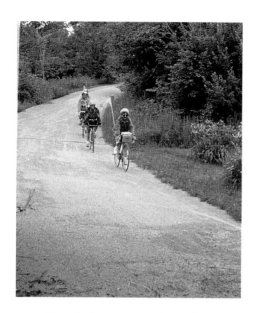

Exercise is an opportunity to give your mind a break.

and dancing crazily to hyper music. Aerobic exercise is so named because your muscles use up oxygen as fast as they get it. Walking, jogging, cycling, cross-country skiing and swimming are all aerobic exercise. They also give your psyche a boost, giving you a chance to clear your mind or sort through problems. Exercise is a great way to relax, providing an outlet for all that pent-up stress we talked about in Chapter 1. Exercise also triggers production of a natural pain reliever in the form of endorphins, known in some circles as "runner's high." This accounts for some people's seeming addiction to their exercise routine. Only in extreme cases is this "addiction" something to worry about. Generally, you'll grow to depend on your workout for the mental down-time.

3 *Balance Your Diet*

While the food at spas can vary from very health-conscious to not so heart-friendly, the general notion of spa cuisine is low-fat. Interesting flavors are achieved through seasonings that use fresh herbs and natural food juices, instead of rich sauces loaded with butter fat. Changing to and maintaining healthy "spa-style" habits starts in the supermarket. Follow these basic tips when choosing products from the four main food groups and you can't go wrong:

FRUITS AND VEGETABLES Aside from olives and avocados, which are high in fat, anything goes with this food group. Fresh is the most nutritious choice, followed by frozen (without sugar, salt or sauces). Canned products are usually high in sugar or sodium, and the canning process sometimes destroys nutrients. Eating dried fruit can contribute to tooth decay. Whole fruits and the peels of vegetables (both well washed) add fiber and extra nutrients to your diet. Cook fruits and vegetables minimally, or eat them raw for maximum nutritional value.

Requirements—At least four servings of approximately one-half cup daily. Include one good Vitamin C source (for example, citrus fruit)

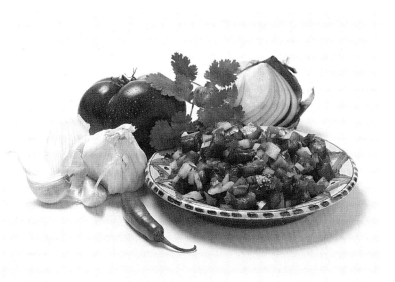

*Fruits and vegetables are excellent
sources of Vitamins A and C.*

each day. Frequently include deep yellow (for example, squash) or
dark green vegetables for Vitamin A. Choose high-fiber vegetables
such as broccoli, cauliflower and carrots.

Decrease added butter, margarine, creams and sauces and coconut.

Increase fresh, frozen, canned (avoid heavy syrups), and dried fruits
and vegetables.

Go easy on avocados and olives.

BREADS AND CEREALS Choose whole-grain, unrefined or fortified products from this group. Whole-wheat bread that is
stone-ground preserves the nutrients that steel grinding destroys.
Cereals should be unrefined and without sugar. Choose whole-wheat
pastas and crackers and brown rice. Popcorn (air-popped) is a nutritious, low-calorie snack that is high in fiber (but don't overload the
butter). Wheat germ and bran can be sneaked into muffin recipes or
sprinkled on top of cereal or yogurt. Avoid bread and cereal products
made with palm or coconut oil.

Requirements—At least four servings daily (a serving equals one
slice of bread; one ounce of ready-to-eat cereal; one-half to three-

EXPERIMENT WITH FOOD SUBSTITUTIONS

There are more and more cookbooks available today emphasizing low-fat recipes. But if you're working from older recipes, butter and cream may be high on the list of ingredients. Rich creamy sauces are not verboten in a healthy diet. But there are some improvements you can make to keep the fat low and flavor high. Where table or whipping cream is called for, try plain low-fat yogurt or 2% milk. Switch from regular butter to low-fat butter or soya margarine, and try lighter oils such as safflower or peanut instead of vegetable. Olive oil, which is a neutral fat, has been shown to have positive benefits for the cardiovascular system. A mixture of safflower and olive oil is a healthy choice.

We are lucky to have a wide variety of foods to choose from in our supermarkets. Here's a list of healthier options:

- low-sodium soy sauce instead of regular soy sauce
- farmer's cheese instead of cream cheese
- non-fat plain yogurt with added fruit or unsweetened conserve instead of sweetened yogurt
- raspberry or pear vinegar instead of salad dressing
- low-sodium crisp or flatbread-type crackers instead of salty, high-fat crackers
- tuna packed in water instead of oil
- whole-wheat or vegetable pasta instead of bleached white pasta
- whole-wheat stone-ground bread instead of white bread
- unsweetened fruit-only conserves instead of jams or jellies

quarters cup of cooked cereal, grits, cornmeal, rice or pasta of any kind; a half a bagel, English muffin, roll, tortilla or muffin; two rice, corn or wheat cakes; three cups of air-popped corn; one-half cup of cooked peas or corn. Whole grains or enriched breads and cereals are a rich source of B vitamins and fiber.

Decrease greasy rolls and muffins, egg noodles and pasta, egg bagels and bread, croissants.

Increase whole-grain breads and cereals (oatmeal, oat bran, whole wheat, wheat bran, rye), rice, pasta noodles (with no added fat).

Go easy on muffins and quick breads.

DAIRY PRODUCTS Calcium is an essential mineral for healthy bones, and the main source is dairy products. If you can't stand milk, make sure you supplement your diet with low-fat or part-skim cheese and low-fat yogurt. If you still guzzle two or three glasses of milk a day, consider switching to a 1% or skim milk. Try ice milk or sorbet instead of ice cream. Dairy products also include protein, riboflavin and Vitamins A, B_6 and B_{12}. Milk is often fortified with Vitamin D to assist in calcium absorption. Dairy foods must be monitored in cholesterol-restricted diets.

Requirements

Children under 9 years of age	2 to 3 servings a day
Children, 9 to 12	3 servings a day
Teens	4 servings a day
Adults, male and female	2 servings a day
Pregnant women	3 servings a day
Nursing mothers	4 servings a day

A serving equals any of the following: one eight-ounce cup of milk, one cup of plain yogurt, two one-inch cubes of cheese, two ounces processed cheese food, one and a half cups ice cream or ice milk, four tablespoons or four ounces Parmesan cheese, two cups cottage cheese.

Decrease whole milk (regular, evaporated, condensed), whole milk cheese, whole milk cottage cheese (4%), ice cream, whole milk yogurt, imitation milk products, most non-dairy creamers, whipped toppings.

Increase skim or 1% milk—liquid, powdered, evaporated; non-fat yogurt; skim milk cheese; low-fat cottage cheese (1% or 2%); farmer or pot cheese; ice milk; buttermilk made from skim milk.

Go easy on 2% milk, part skim cheese, low-fat yogurt.

MEAT, FISH, POULTRY AND BEANS Although the fat is what gives meat its flavor, stick to the lean cuts. Chicken, turkey and fish are good low-fat choices, but shrimp is high in cholesterol. Choose tuna packed in water, not oil, and check for salt and fat content in all

MAKE SURE YOU'RE GETTING ENOUGH VITAMINS AND MINERALS

Most nutritionists agree that if you eat a well-balanced diet and follow a healthy lifestyle in general, vitamin pills are largely unnecessary. However, individuals affected by the following conditions may be helped by sensible vitamin supplementation.

- People on low-cal diets (under 1,200 calories) who may not be able to get all the vitamins they need each day
- Pregnant or breast-feeding women
- Seniors whose slower metabolism requires they get the same amount of nutrition from fewer calories
- People suffering from certain conditions such as alcoholism or anemia, for example, whose bodies cannot store vitamins as well

Check with your health-care professional if you feel you will benefit from vitamin supplementation.

CHOLESTEROL

Blood cholesterol is the naturally occurring cholesterol produced by the liver. There are two types: good, high-density lipoproteins known as HDLs and bad, low-density lipoproteins known as LDLs. Everyone has these two types, but the ratio varies. A higher ratio of HDL to LDL means less risk of heart disease. Aerobic exercise increases the ratio of HDL to LDL, as does decreasing the amount of cholesterol and saturated fats you eat.

High blood cholesterol is a genetic predisposition, so if it runs in your family, there's a good chance you could have it too. The appropriate level depends on age and sex. High risk factors include, besides family history, cigarette smoking, high blood pressure, low level of HDL, diabetes, history of strokes or blockage of blood vessels in other body parts, and severe obesity. Men with at least one of these risk factors, and women with at least two, must take special precautions to guard their health.

	United States	Canada
Healthy	0–200 milligrams per decaliter	0–5.2 millimoles per liter
Caution	201–239	5.2–6.2
High Risk	240+	6.2+

Note: Measurements are for those thirty years of age and over.

prepared fish and meats. Peanut butter and other nuts and seeds are high in fat, as well as protein. Eggs also fall into this category, and their versatility and low-cal content makes them a good food choice. However, the yolks are high in cholesterol (the bad kind) and they are usually accompanied by fatty bacon and greasy potatoes. Most egg dishes can be prepared with half the yolks the recipe specifies or even no yolks. Crepes, quiches, omelettes and fritattas make elegant dishes and usually call for vegetables instead of home fries.

Foods in this group are high in protein, phosphorus, Vitamins B_6 and B_{12} and other vitamins and minerals, but only foods of animal origin contain B_{12} naturally. Varying your choices among these foods will maximize the benefits. Dietary cholesterol also occurs only in foods of animal origin. The highest concentration is found in organ meats and egg yolks. Fish and shellfish, except shrimp, are relatively low in dietary cholesterol.

Requirements—Two servings a day. One serving equals two or three ounces of lean, cooked meat, poultry or fish without the bone; one

THE KITCHEN MEDICINE CABINET

Naturopaths have known for centuries that many foods have pharmaceutical properties. The medical community has been slower to catch on but has begun studying many common foods for scientific evidence that they do what people claim.

- Broccoli, cabbage, cauliflower and bok choy have been linked with lower incidence of colorectal cancer.
- Some researchers have found that garlic, onions and leeks have a cholesterol-lowering effect; others have linked high-garlic diets to low rates of death from heart disease and to a lower incidence of stomach cancer.
- Olive oil and canola oil have been found to lower LDLs and raise HDLs.
- Mushrooms and radishes are loaded with selenium, which has been linked to healthy hearts.
- Cranberry juice has been linked to lower rates of urinary tract infections.
- Yogurt (with active cultures) can stimulate immune-system cells that help fight the bacteria that can cause intestinal infections and diarrhea. It also prevents yeast infections and has been shown to slow the development of colon tumors in lab animals.
- Oat bran, flax and other soluble fibers reduce cholesterol.
- Tofu and other soybean products are linked with reduced rates of breast cancer; they are also loaded with phytoestrogens that can provide a natural alternative to hormone replacement therapy for menopausal women.
- Researchers speculate that the high fiber and beta-carotene found in most fruits and vegetables are responsible for reducing the risk of several types of cancer.
- Warm milk has an active ingredient, tryptophan, that really does help get you to sleep.

egg; one-half to three-quarters of a cup of cooked beans, peas, soybeans or lentils; two tablespoons of peanut butter; one-quarter to one-half cup of nuts or seeds. Calories vary depending on fat content.

Decrease egg yolks—no more than three or four a week; organ meats; fatty red meats, such as beef, lamb, pork; cold cuts; sausage, hot dogs and bacon; spare ribs; canned meats, meat mixtures; duck.

FOOD PREPARATION TIPS

- Avoid convenience foods, including low-cal frozen dinners. Most are high in sodium and lower in nutritional value than freshly made foods.
- Learn to steam vegetables.
- Broil and bake meats, fish and poultry.
- Eat whole-grain pastas with primavera and marinara sauces.
- Make a simple meal plan based on the requirements from the four food groups, and write out a shopping list from your plan. Stroll the grocery store aisles with a purposeful list, instead of haphazardly filling your cart with whatever looks good or is marked down, which usually results in a heftier bill, and a heftier you.

Increase poultry without skin, all fish, egg whites (two whites equal one whole egg in recipes), dried beans, lean cuts of beef or pork or veal (no more than two or three times a week), tofu.

Go easy on nuts and nut butters.

FATS, ALCOHOL AND SUGAR GROUPS This is not an official food group, but given we eat so much food from it, it bears mentioning. Concentrate on getting adequate amounts of the nutrient-rich foods in the other categories before resorting to this group to meet your daily energy needs.

This group includes butter, margarine, mayonnaise, salad dressings, lard, oil and all other fats, candy, sugar, jam, jelly, syrup, soft drinks, cocoa, pastry, cookies, cake, pie and all other sweets, and alcoholic beverages. Also included are all refined but unenriched breads and flour products. Foods from these groups are not recommended, so there is no defined serving size. With the exception of vegetable oils, these foods consist of empty calories. Vegetable oils supply Vitamin E and essential fatty acids. The caloric content of carbohydrates and proteins is four calories per gram. Alcohol has seven calories per gram and fats have nine calories per gram.

Decrease butter, mayonnaise, margarine, hydrogenated fats, shortening, chocolate, coconut oil, palm oil, lard, bacon fat, sour cream, cream cheese, cream, half-and-half, most non-dairy creamers, regular salad dressing, gravies and cream sauces.

Increase chicken or vegetable broth for sautéing, apple butter, natural jams, mustard, non-fat yogurt, low-fat cottage cheese, low-fat ricotta cheese, tofu, no-oil salad dressing.

Go easy on reduced-fat sour cream or cream cheese, diet margarine, creamy diet salad dressings, diet mayonnaise.

Food doesn't make you fat; your behaviors, attitudes, and choices make you fat.

—*Thelma Wayler, Green Mountain at Fox Run, Vermont*

4 *Examine Your Eating Behavior*

Much of our inability to lose weight has little to do with what we eat, but lots to do with how we eat. On the run, in front of the television, quick mouthfuls between kids' meals—all interfere with your body's ability to metabolize food properly. Some habits simply lead to overeating. Try the following guidelines:

- Measure portions, then take only one.
- Put leftovers away immediately.
- Eat slowly, taking 20 minutes or more to finish the main course.
- Pace yourself by putting your utensils down between bites and taking a break.
- If you're full, don't feel compelled to clean your plate, despite what your mother may have told you.
- Start drinking 1% or skim milk.
- In restaurants, ration the bread and butter before the main course is served.
- Meals should have their own time and place. Don't make a habit out of eating at your desk, in the car, or in front of the television.

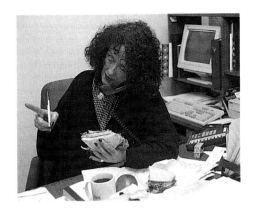

Examine your eating behavior carefully—lifelong habits may be preventing you from obtaining your optimal weight.

5 Drink Lots of Water

Besides incorporating foods from all four food groups, you must remember to drink lots of water to wash it all down. Water is a key component of all the energy reactions in the body, and it also transports nutrients and removes wastes. Without adequate water in your system, you function at less than peak performance.

Most people are underhydrated most of the time without realizing it. Your thirst is not a good indication of your fluid needs. Aim for six to eight 8-ounce glasses of fluid per day, which includes milk, fruit juice and vegetable juice, but not soft drinks or caffeinated beverages. Caffeine, in particular, dehydrates the body, so limit its intake.

It is important to keep your fluids up before, during and after a physical workout. Thirst is an unreliable gauge of impending dehydration because you can tolerate a water loss equaling 5% of your body weight before thirst demands you drink.

Drink two cups of water before exercising, one cup every 20 minutes while exercising and two cups beyond thirst requirements after

TIPS FOR KICKING THE JUNK FOOD HABIT

- Pay attention to the labels—most chips and crackers now come in low-sodium versions at the same price. But don't make it an excuse to eat more.
- Don't deprive your sweet tooth. Instead, pick a weekly time to indulge. For example, every Wednesday lunch is followed by a chocolate bar.
- Pretzels and popcorn are lower in fat than potato chips.
- Try pizza without the fatty pepperoni and sausage, but with peppers, onions, mushrooms and tomatoes instead.

THE GARDEN MEDICINE CABINET

Plants are the original source of most of the drugs we use today, although today's drugs are now synthetically produced to save money. Using essential oils is one way to access these curative properties (see aromatherapy, page 90), but the ground flowers, seeds, leaves and roots, mixed into tinctures, poultices or washes, have their own medicinal effect. Turn your patch of earth into a mini-pharmacy with some of these time-honored herbal remedies (but be sure of your horticultural identification skills first):

- Make a compress of ground basil leaves and water to relieve headaches and anxiety. Crushed leaves are also good on insect bites or stings.
- The ground leaves of bay laurel steeped in water relieve the pain of rheumatism as well as sprains and bruises. Also makes a good antiseptic.
- Crushed chamomile flowers and leaves mixed with water or alcohol make a soothing compress for wounds, burns and swellings.
- The leaves and flowers of clary sage mixed with alcohol make an all-purpose astringent good for general skin care.
- Cowslip flowers and leaves mixed with flaxseed or coconut oil can be used to treat burns.
- A dandelion root tincture calms acne and skin eruptions.
- A fresh evening primrose plant chopped and mixed in water makes an effective wash for minor wounds and skin eruptions.
- Stir fennel seeds in boiling water and let cool slightly for a powerful disinfectant and anti-inflammatory wash.
- Geranium leaves ground in water can be used to treat scar tissue, inflammation, eczema, shingles and acne. The mixture also makes a cooling compress for engorged breasts.
- Boil juniper berries and needles in water to make an antiseptic cleanser good for soothing minor wounds, rheumatism, pulled muscles and bruises.
- Ground licorice root mixed with water reduces redness of the skin and soothes eczema and psoriasis.
- Crushed flowers and leaves of the savory plant, mixed with water, make a refreshing gargle and keep athlete's foot at bay.
- Thyme leaves and flowers stirred into boiling water have a germicidal effect, good for foot soaks and treating dandruff.

your workout. If you have had caffeinated liquids or alcohol within 12 hours of exercising, drink an extra glass of water. This will also help your kidneys eliminate the inherent toxins. Water intake will also help reduce body temperature while exercising your body sweats it out: remember, the body absorbs cold drinks faster than hot ones.

6 Order Carefully in Restaurants

It isn't always easy, but it is possible to eat healthy, low-fat meals in restaurants. It takes careful, conscientious ordering, limiting portions and, sometimes, special requests.

EATING HEALTHY WHILE EATING OUT

Restaurant	First Choice	Second Choice	Worst Choice
Steakhouse	Lean Cuts **Best prepared:** grilled, i.e., London broil, filet mignon, sirloin	Broiled top or bottom round, flank or sirloin tip, i.e., Porterhouse, rib steak or rib roast	Anything fried. Also avoid roasted organ meats, fatty cuts and T-bones
Seafood	Halibut, whitefish, flounder swordfish or bluefish **Best prepared:** in white wine or lemon juice, stewed, broiled or baked	Scallops, lobster, mackerel, snapper, salmon or sardines	Shimp and anything breaded, deep-fried or prepared with butter or cream sauces
Chinese/Thai	Chicken, fish, or vegetable dishes **Best prepared:** in clear chicken broth, with garlic, scallions, vegetables or ginger sauce	Beef or shellfish	Duck or pork. Avoid brown bean sauce, soy sauce, peanuts, oyster sauce, sweet and sour sauce and cream sauce
Italian	Chicken, fish, veal or pasta entrées **Best prepared:** in wine, or with tomatoes, mushrooms, onions or lemon. Marinara and primavera sauces are good	Shellfish, beef, pork or sausage	Avoid butter, oil, anchovies, fried or breaded dishes. Also avoid meat and cream sauces and anything prepared Parmigiana
Japanese	Raw (sushi) or cooked fish	Chicken or beef	Duck or pork. Limit soy sauce, tempura style or sukiyaki
French	Veal, fish, chicken or frog legs **Best prepared:** with tomato sauce, mushrooms, garlic, vegetables, brown sauce or grapes	Shellfish, lamb, ham or pork	Brains, liver, sweetbreads, duck or goose. Avoid cheese, butter, almonds, cherry or orange sauce, breading, cream or Hollandaise sauce, or bacon
Mexican	Chicken, vegetable or bean dishes **Best prepared:** with onions, sherry, garlic, tomatoes or peppers		Avoid butter, cheese, oil, sour cream, chocolate and nuts

Many of today's drugs are based on ancient herbal remedies.

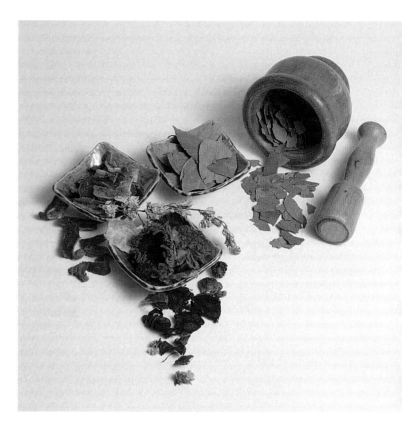

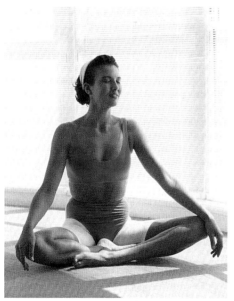

Yoga helps improve balance and flexibility.

7 Learn to Stretch

The days of feel-it-burn aerobics classes are long gone. Today, people are recognizing that their souls need a workout as much as their bodies. The following activities combine stretching, breathing and visualization to achieve a peaceful state of mind. Benefits include better sleep, which helps reduce stress, increased flexibility and relieved muscle tension.

- Yoga—A good yoga workout lasts about an hour and a half. After a warm-up, an instructor guides you through a series of "postures" or intensive stretches that you can later do on your own at home. Each posture is held for about 30 seconds. Yoga emphasizes balance—both physical and mental—and also increases flexibility.

- T'ai Chi—The ancient Chinese art looks so peaceful and serene, but make no mistake, it's a workout. A t'ai chi set can

WHAT ABOUT VEGETARIANISM?

The strong links between animal fat and many cancers and heart disease have prompted many people to cut red meat out of their diets. Some, for moral reasons as well, have given up poultry. Lactovegetarians include milk in their diets; ovolactovegetarians include milk and eggs. Vegans include neither. Fish is allowed in most vegetarian, but not vegan, diets.

A totally vegetarian diet must be carefully planned to compensate for the missing protein, Vitamin B_{12}, calcium, riboflavin and iron provided by lean meats and dairy products. Here are some tips:

- Select a wide variety of plant foods in order to obtain the spectrum of important nutrients.
- Minimize the consumption of empty-calorie "junk" foods and maintain calorie intake at appropriate levels.
- Replace meat with increased intake of legumes, soy products and nuts, and, if eating a lactovegetarian diet, low-fat milk and milk products.
- Increase whole-grain cereals and products.
- Vegans must replace the nutrients found in milk. Fortified soybean milk can be used and B_{12} supplements may be necessary.
- Plan meals carefully using the four vegetarian food groups: fruits and vegetables (4+ servings per day); breads and cereals (4+ servings per day); milk or soy milk (2 cups or more per day); legumes, nut, meat analogs (2 cups or more per day).

To compensate for the missing amino acids found in animal proteins, you have to combine "incomplete" proteins of plant foods. Try a little food math:

Rice + beans, nuts, wheat germ, dairy products or eggs = complete protein

Beans + corn, rice, dairy products, nuts, grains or eggs = complete protein

Pasta + spinach, wheat germ, dairy products or eggs = complete protein

Vegetables + nuts, rice, sunflower seeds, wheat germ, dairy or eggs = complete protein

Vegans must eat dark green vegetables and nuts for calcium; fortified soybean milk, meat analogs such as tofu, or vitamin supplements for B_{12}; whole and enriched grain and cereal products for riboflavin and iron (increase iron absorption by including an ascorbic acid source such as broccoli in the meal). Vegans should have their blood iron levels checked periodically.

consist of between 21 and 254 moves. They are deliberate, precise positions that demand focus and concentration from the participant. The goal is to relax muscles and prevent spine shrinkage with age.

- Pilates—Named for its inventor Joseph Pilates (pronounced Pee-lah-tees), this innovative stretching technique is taking over the home gyms of Hollywood. Done on the floor or in a series of specially designed contraptions, Pilates focuses on lining up the vertical and horizontal planes of the body. The moves are more flowing and dance-like than the positions of yoga and t'ai chi. The aim is longer, leaner muscles that operate at peak efficiency.

- Gardening—Perhaps it was Jane Fonda who first made the connection between gardening and fitness when she described one of her exercises as "pull those weeds, pull those weeds!" You'd never consider gardening an aerobic activity, but it is an ideal place to stretch your legs and arms. Like yoga and t'ai chi, gardening also has an element of serenity, providing you with a time to collect your thoughts.
- Ballroom Dancing—It's definitely in again, thanks to increasing interest in ballroom dancing as a competitive sport (witness the rise of ice dancing, too). Ballroom dancing has the added benefit of combining exercise with a night on the town. One hour of vigorous dancing is roughly equivalent to walking 17 miles.
- The Therapy Ball—Known as an exercise ball or therapy ball because physiotherapists often use it to help stroke patients recover, this large rubber ball provides a body-friendly way to stretch and tone. Simply sitting and balancing on the ball requires you to coordinate all muscles from the soles of your feet to the top of your spine. Lie on the ball, on your front or back, to tighten flabby abs, or lie sideways over it to stretch your oblique abdominals. The possibilities are endless.

8 Design a Fitness Program That's Right for You

Although you can luxuriate all day long in a hot tub if you want, spa guests are encouraged to participate in weight training, yoga, aerobics, swimming, tennis, hiking … some spas even offer snowshoeing excursions for the more adventurous set.

Exercise can be divided into four categories:
- cardiovascular, the ability to take in, transport and utilize oxygen;
- flexibility, the range of motion about a joint;

- muscular strength, the force a muscle or muscle group can exert against a resistance;
- and muscular endurance, the ability of a muscle group to exert force or maintain a degree of force over a long period of time.

CARDIOVASCULAR ENDURANCE   Aerobic activities using large major muscle groups are the best ones to improve cardiovascular endurance. The physiological benefits are myriad:

- strengthens heart muscle;
- enlarges main heart chamber allowing more blood pumped per beat;
- lowers resting heart rate;
- increases ability to do more work at prescribed target heart-rate range (see page 51);
- increases collateral circulation (branching blood vessels off main blood vessels);
- increases body's ability to use fat as a fuel source.

Cardio exercise also has several health benefits:
- decreases risk of heart disease;
- may help lower blood pressure;
- decreases percentage of body fat;
- may help lower risk for osteoporosis;
- may help control or reduce risk for diabetes;
- increases lung volume;
- improves emotional well-being;
- increases self-confidence, self-esteem and self-image;
- improves quality of sleep;
- creates higher levels of energy.

FLEXIBILITY   Your flexibility is limited by bone, muscle, ligaments, tendons, connective tissue and skin. Greater flexibility not only enhances how well you perform certain skills and activities, but it is also often prescribed for prevention and rehabilitation of some muscular injuries, lower-back pain, muscular tension and soreness.

You can safely improve flexibility with static stretching exercises, in which muscles are gradually stretched without bouncing or forcing. Assume a mild stretched position (see sketches on pages 47–48) and hold it for 20 to 30 seconds. Focus on the muscle group being exercised, and remember to keep breathing. (Holding your breath makes you too tense to appreciate the stretch.) Stretching to increase flexibility is most effective after a workout when the muscles are warm, but stretching should also be a part of your warm-up phase to prepare the muscles for action.

TOTAL BODY STRETCH

Stretching increases flexibility and decreases the risk of injury, reduces muscle soreness, and just feels great! Move slowly and gently while doing stretches. Don't push too far—it should not hurt. Stretch to the point where you feel resistance, then relax, breathe deeply, and hold for 30 to 60 seconds or more.

Start in the **Fundamental Stance**. Stand with your toes pointing forward and your feet planted at least shoulder width apart. Your weight should be distributed evenly between both feet and your arms should be at your sides. Keep your knees relaxed—never lock them!—and hold your abdominal muscles in.

Breathe and Stretch Take a breath and begin to lift your arms out from your sides, then up over your head. Exhale and push your arms out and down. Feel the stretch in your arms and shoulders. Repeat five times.

Head Isolation Turn your head to the left, slowly and gently. Be sure to move your head only. Return to center and then turn your head to the right. Repeat several times for both sides. Now tilt your head to the left, keeping your chin centered, until your ear almost reaches your left shoulder. Feel this stretch in the right side of your neck. Reverse sides and repeat several times.

Shoulder Isolation Lift your shoulders up toward your ears several times. Roll both shoulders forward, down, and back, in one gentle, continuous motion. Keep the rest of your body still. Repeat five times, then reverse direction of roll.

Shoulder Pull Clasp your hands behind your back and press your elbows toward each other. Holding your hands behind your tailbone, bend forward gently, lifting your clasped hands up and pressing your shoulder blades together.

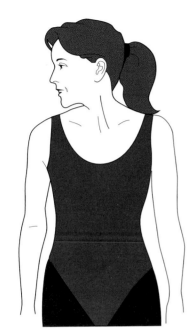

Head isolation

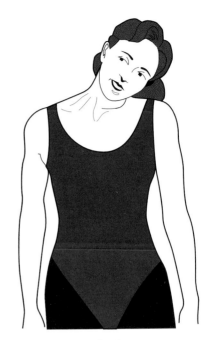

Head isolation

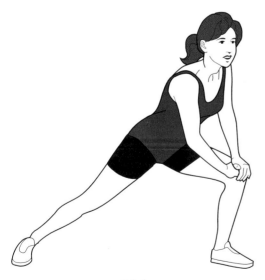

Side lunge

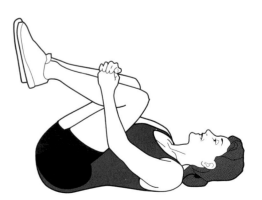

Lower back stretch

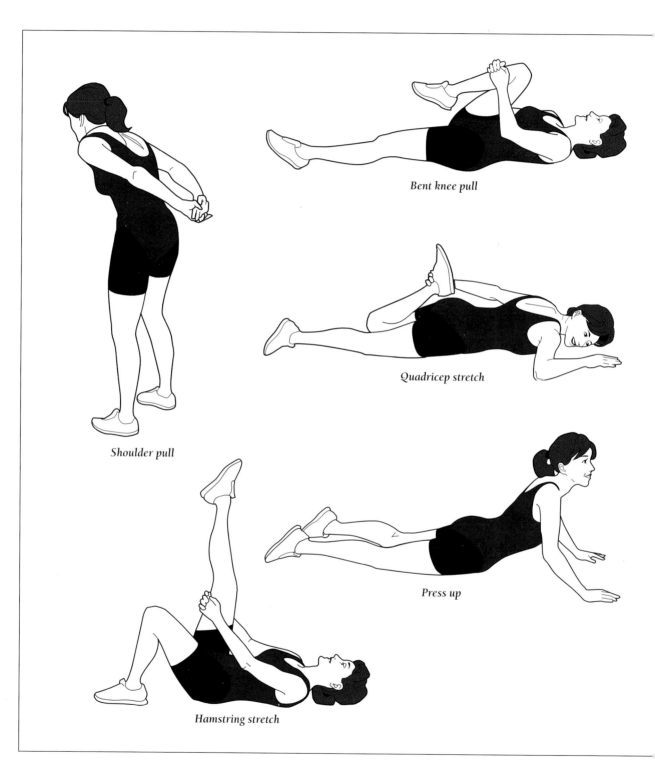

Bent knee pull

Quadricep stretch

Shoulder pull

Press up

Hamstring stretch

Waist Bends Place your hands on your hips, elbows pointed out. Keeping your lower body still, bend to the right. Relax and feel the stretch on the left side of your torso. Repeat on the left side.

Half Knee Bends Keeping your spine in alignment, slowly bend your knees and lower hips. Keep your heels firmly planted on the floor. Slowly push back up, taking care to keep your knees directly in line with your toes, your weight evenly distributed, and your spine long. Don't bend forward or arch your back. Repeat five times. Repeat this stretch with your toes turned out a little and feel it in your inner and outer thighs and calf muscles.

Side Lunge Shift your weight to your left leg and let your right leg slide out as you bend your left knee. Keep your knee directly in line with your toes. Place both hands on your knee and, bending forward, feel the stretch in your left thigh. Turn your toes out a little, keeping your knee in line with your toes, and feel the stretch in your groin area. Reverse sides and repeat.

Calf Stretch Place your hands on your hips, then lunge forward with your weight on your left leg and your right leg stretched out behind you. Keep your left knee bent and in line with your toes. Both heels should be on the floor, both knees relaxed. Feel the stretch in your right calf. Now bend your right knee more, still keeping your heel on the floor. Feel the stretch lower in your calf. Reverse legs and repeat.

Ankle Rotation Holding on to something stable, lift your ankle and slowly perform a complete circle five times. Repeat, circling in the opposite direction. Switch ankles and repeat entire cycle. This can also be done while sitting in a chair.

These remaining stretches are performed lying down on the floor. Use a mat whenever possible.

Lower Back Stretch Lie on your back with your legs bent and your feet flat on the floor. Slowly bring both knees to your chest and clasp your arms around your legs. Hold for several seconds, then release. Repeat five times.

Bent Knee Pull Lie on your back with your legs extended. Bring your right knee to your chest while keeping your left leg, lower back, and head pressed to the floor. Hold for several seconds, then release. Reverse legs and repeat.

Hamstring Stretch Lie on your back, with your knees bent and your feet flat on the floor. Bring your right knee up to your chest. Clasping your hands behind your knee, slowly straighten your leg to the ceiling. If you can't straighten your leg, then press your knee back a bit toward your other foot. Hold for several seconds, then release. Repeat with other leg.

Press Up Lie face down with your legs slightly apart. Bend your arms, with your elbows next to your ribs and your palms flat on the floor next to your shoulders. Slowly and gently lift your head, neck, shoulders, and upper torso off the floor by straightening your elbows. Only lift yourself as far as is comfortable. Hold for several seconds, then release slowly. Repeat five times.

Quadriceps Stretch Lie face down, with your head and shoulders relaxed on the floor. Bend your left knee and try to grasp your left foot with your left hand. If you can hold on to the foot or ankle easily, gently pull your foot and hold for several seconds. Keep your knee in line with your shoulder at all times. Reverse to your right side and repeat. You might find this easier lying on your side.

MUSCULAR STRENGTH Strength is developed using progressive resistance exercises that "overload" the muscle groups. Choose a weight you can lift no more than about eight to ten times—each lift is known as a repetition. Strength gains can occur with a single set (eight to ten repetitions); however, multiple sets (three to six) with minute-long rest periods in between have been shown to make you stronger, faster. The best way to build muscular strength is by using free weights or weight training machines. However, you can increase resistance while swimming, for example, by using hand paddles or webbed gloves to pull more water. Or try using wrist weights while running.

MUSCULAR ENDURANCE Programs of high repetition and low resistance—two to three sets of anything over 12 repetitions, at an easier weight—is the best way to build muscular endurance. Exercises specifically addressing muscular endurance are recommended in order to improve performance in specific sports, to enhance body

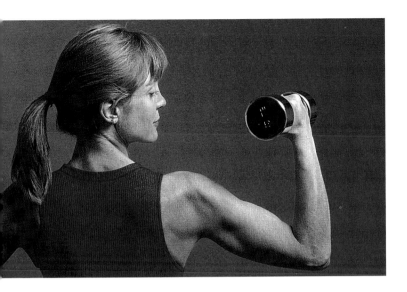

Weight training with free weights or weight machines builds muscular strength.

posture control and to help prevent injury. Free weights, weight training machines, calisthenics/body contour exercises on land or in the water and aerobic exercise all help build muscular endurance.

In the same way that a healthy diet combines food selections from all four food groups, a healthy exercise program combines exercises from all four categories. Although you might be able to run long distances with ease, if you neglect strength training, your overall fitness suffers. Likewise, an avid golfer might be able to drive a ball 200 yards, but may get winded running to the clubhouse from a sudden shower.

Ideally, you should exercise every day. Whether that's a swim at the Y or an aerobics class at the local gym is up to you. But adopt a program that you enjoy. If you find aerobics painful on your joints, don't persist. Try a rowing machine or a low-impact class. If you're not a particularly good swimmer, you're probably not going to benefit from 40 laps the way you should. If you're set on pool exercise, try your hand at aquafitness—aerobics in the water.

No matter the exercise you undertake, the session must include:

- a warm-up—three to five minutes of gentle stretching and cardio exercise that gets the heart pumping, such as marching or jogging on the spot. A good warm-up will gradually increase blood flow and temperature of the muscles, stimulate heart

FIGURING OUT YOUR TARGET HEART RATE

To determine if you're exercising at a sufficient pace, monitor your heart rate. Place your first two fingers on your wrist or the hollow of your neck. Count the number of pulses in a 10-second period, then multiply that number by six for your heart rate (heart beats per minute). The goal is to increase your heart rate. For your estimated target heart rate, subtract half your age from 220 (for women). Multiply that number by 65 percent for the minimum exercising heart rate, and by 75 percent for the maximum. (See chart on page 52.) If you're just starting an exercise regime, don't push yourself past the lower end of your target. Building aerobic strength takes time. An easier way to determine if you're going too fast is to take the simple talk test. If you're too winded to carry on a conversation, you're working too hard.

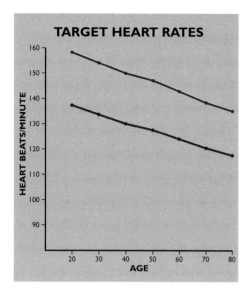

TARGET HEART RATES

and lungs, stretch muscles and tendons to prepare for more forceful contractions, act as a precaution against unnecessary injuries and muscle soreness, and prepare you mentally.

- a conditioning period—the main focus of the session. Aerobic and muscular endurance exercises should be done for at least 20 to 45 minutes each session (in your target heart range for cardio exercises) at least three to five days a week. Muscular strength conditioning should be done every other day.

- a cool-down—eight to fifteen minutes of gradually reducing the demands on the heart and lungs, decreasing the blood flow to the muscles and shunting the blood back to the heart and internal organs. Stretching (five to ten minutes) is also an important aspect of the cool-down. Studies have shown the greatest improvements in flexibility are achieved in the cool-down period when the muscles are warm.

TYPES OF EXERCISES The most important component of physical fitness is cardiorespiratory fitness. Good aerobic activities include brisk walking, running, swimming, cycling, hiking, stair climbing, rowing, cross-country skiing, jump rope, aerobic dance and mini-trampoline work. Racquet sports are not recommended to attain cardiovascular fitness, but may be a reasonable means to help maintain conditioning.

FREQUENCY OF EXERCISE A good exercise program is a consistent program. Someone in average physical condition should exercise at least three days a week. If you're in good physical condition, you can exercise more often—up to six or even seven days a week. Increase frequency gradually to minimize risk of injury while you're developing stamina. That sounds like a lot of exercise, but doing a little bit each day allows you to build it into your daily routine in smaller intervals of a half hour to an hour. And once you get in the habit of taking that lunch-hour fitness class, for example, you'll be hooked. If channel surfing has been your main exercise for too long, you may have to exercise for short periods several times a day until you're in better shape.

LENGTH OF EXERCISE SESSION An exercise session should be long enough to burn about 300 calories. Typically, 20 minutes is the minimum and 45 to 50 minutes is the ceiling for cardiovascular conditioning. It depends on intensity, too—running three miles at an eight-minute-per-mile pace (24 minutes) will take less time than walking three miles at a 15-minute-per-mile pace (45 minutes). After one hour, the cardio benefits diminish considerably the longer you go; however, the calorie-burning continues. Activities of a more intermittent nature, such as singles tennis or racquetball, may require up to 90 minutes to equal the benefit of more continuous activities.

INTENSITY The exercise must be intense enough to get your heart rate up into its target range (see chart on page 52), but not so hard as to have the risks exceed the benefits. Learning to "listen" to your own body can be quite helpful in establishing the proper level. Remember, exercising shouldn't be painful beyond the point of discomfort to be effective.

9 *Set up a Home Gym*

Some people love the social aspects of working out, but can't quite seem to find the time or motivation to get to the gym. Others may enjoy outdoor workouts but find that inclement weather thwarts their best intentions. One way to make daily workouts easier is to invest in some equipment for a home gym. Whether you favor the low-tech ease of a jump rope or the high-tech gadgetry of a weight machine, there is a perfect home gym for you.

But before you reach for your credit card and order the latest abdominal cruncher-sizer from a TV infomercial, consider the type of exercise you like to do. Do you like repetition, or do you bore easily? Do you respond well to physical challenges, or prefer not to feel like you're struggling? Then, of course, you have to consider your environment. Where will you be setting up your home gym? Do you have a separate room, like a basement or spare bedroom, or will you be working in the middle of the living room? In the case of the latter situation, you'll want portable and compact equipment that stores easily.

STAND TALLER

- Many women often ignore their upper bodies when working out, for fear they will become too muscled in their shoulders, biceps and triceps. Don't make this mistake. Upper body strength is key to having healthy chest strength and good posture, particularly in large-breasted women. A note of caution, however. When you exercise your pectoral muscles, you should also exercise your back—the corresponding opposite muscles.

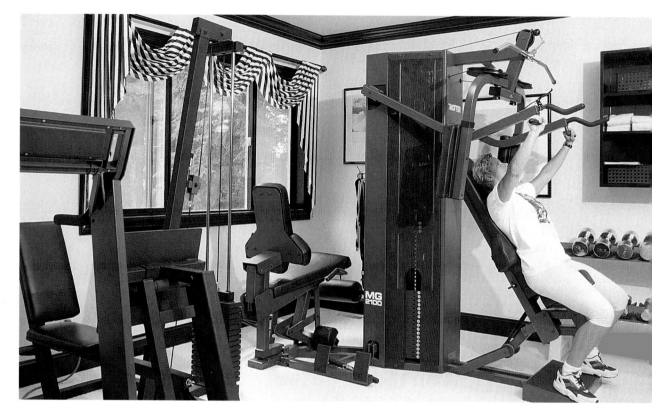

Working out at home is the perfect solution for time-constrained fitness enthusiasts.

In any case, there are some basics you'll probably want:

- a foam rubber mat to make the floor more inviting for flexibility training;
- a set of free weights and a book or video instructing how best to use them;
- access to a stereo if you like to work out to music, and a television if you plan to follow video instruction;
- a watch or clock with a second hand to monitor your heart rate;
- a full-length mirror to check positions and show results.

Benefit	High-Tech	Low-Tech
Cardio	Stationary bike	Stationary adapter for real bike
	Rowing machine	Jump rope
	StairMaster	Reebok step
Strength	Multi-station weight machine	Resistance bands or bar

Stationary bicycles can range in price from $100 to $600. The more expensive models feature electronic measurement devices that can track heart rate and calories burned and intricate flywheel systems that adjust pedal resistance. To achieve aerobic benefit from cycling, you must exercise within your target heart range (see chart on page 52) for 20 to 30 minutes at least three times a week. Many indoor cyclists like to ride while reading or watching television to prevent boredom.

Rowing machines use the large muscles in the legs, as well as the arms, back and abdomen. A good rowing machine costs anywhere from $300 to $600. The best rower uses a cable or flywheel action for resistance rather than a hydraulic piston. Pulling against the cable gives a much smoother action and more closely simulates rowing in water. If you have back problems, consult your physician or chiropractor before beginning a rowing program since some rowing machines—particularly the hydraulic variety—can place excess strain on the back.

Strength-training machines are the best way to progressively "overload" your muscles with increasing amounts of resistance. Free weights are the least expensive solution, but they are not always recommended for the "home" athlete since improper lifting can lead to serious injury. More expensive, but safer, are resistance machines that isolate specific muscle groups. These home gyms range in price from $500 to more than $1,500. "Cable" models that use your own body weight for resistance are generally the least expensive. Multi-station machines (similar to those found in most professional gyms) are the most expensive but do offer a total body workout, and more than one person at a time can use them, too.

DESIGNING THE ROOM If you plan to go all out and dedicate a room in your house to a home gym, there are some features you want to consider. First, decide where your equipment is going to go before you deal with lighting. Make sure you're not casting shadows on television screens or mirrors, and don't be chintzy on wattage. Fluorescent lighting is also preferred over incandescent—it keeps you from getting drowsy and is also a lot more flattering to you (witness the common use of fluorescents in clothing store change rooms). Take advantage of whatever natural light you have. Cardio equipment such as bikes or a StairMaster go best in front of windows, since you're usually on them for a long time and a view is nice.

The walls should be white as darker colors seem to induce sleepiness. A full-length mirror or, even better, a full wall mirror is a good motivator and helps you monitor progress and check your form as you lift, bend or stretch.

Unless you've been blessed with a spare room that isn't loaded with junk, your basement is the most likely place to build a home gym. It's a good choice for eliminating noise and structural hazards, especially the deep ones in newer homes. (Lack of light, however, is a slight disadvantage.) If you plan on installing heavy equipment on a second floor—even a StairMaster—you'll want to put it near the wall to muffle noise. Keep air fresh and circulating with open windows and fans if air-conditioning is out of the question. Ceiling fans are good too, but be aware of their position in low-ceilinged rooms, such as a basement. A typical 15-amp circuit is sufficient for most electric exercise equipment, but if you're not sure about your room's capabilities, hire an electrician to check it out.

10 Start Walking

You don't have to invest in expensive classes, machinery or athletic gear to get a good dose of exercise. Just put on a pair of comfortable shoes and head out the door for a brisk walk. Walking has many advantages:

- It burns body fat.
- It builds muscles. More muscle means you burn more calories at all times, and you can eat more to maintain your weight, or eat the same and lose.
- It builds bone tissue, decreasing the risk of osteoporosis and broken bones.
- It allows you personal time alone, or it can be a social activity with a friend.
- It can be done every day with very little risk of injury or over-training.

BONE UP

- Doctors recommend weight-bearing exercises such as walking, running or tennis to reduce the risk of bone loss, thus preventing osteoporosis.

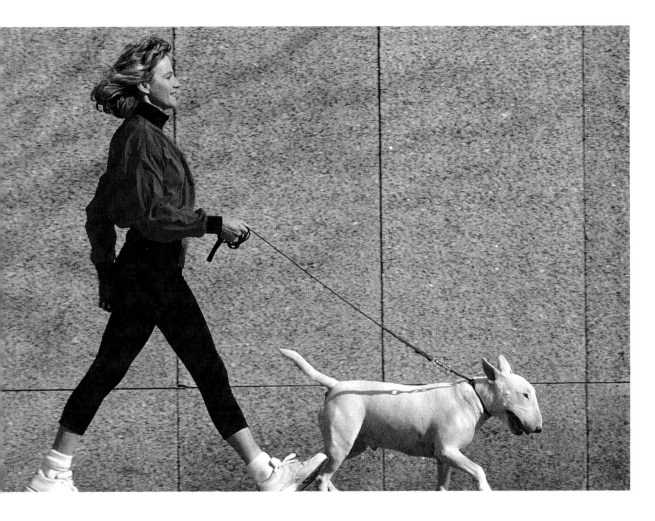

- If you walk at a brisk enough pace, you will exercise your heart muscle to the same degree as in aerobics, with a lot less stress on your body.
- It gets you away from the refrigerator!

Your body burns plenty of calories walking. How much depends on your weight, how far you go, and how fast. But you're not in a race. Set a moderate pace that you can maintain for an hour. You'll burn more fat than walking at a faster speed for less time.

To calculate how many calories you will burn on your walk, divide your weight (in pounds) by 2 to get your base number.

Dog-walking is an excellent way to make exercise part of your daily routine.

FIVE CALORIE BURNERS/ENERGY BOOSTERS

1. Take the stairs—75 calories in five minutes. Alternate climbing two flights with 30 seconds of jogging in place or slower walking down stairs. Gradually increase to 10 sets of two flights each.
2. Walk up hills—45 calories in five minutes. Walk briskly up a moderately steep hill for three minutes, rest 30 seconds and walk slowly down the hill. Repeat three times. Gradually increase to five sets of three-minute climbs. If you have lower-back or knee pain, traverse from side to side as you walk down the hill.
3. Jump rope—85 calories in five minutes. Alternate five sets of 30 jumps with 30 seconds of marching in place. Gradually increase to 10 sets of 50 jumps with 10 seconds of marching in place in between.
4. Walk/run—38 calories in five minutes. Alternate one minute of brisk walking with 30 seconds of easy jogging. Gradually increase to a 1:1 ratio.
5. Stroll—18 calories in five minutes. Walk at a comfortable pace.

- Your base number tells you the number of calories you will burn at a 20-minute-per-mile pace.
- For a 15-minute mile, add 7 calories to the base number.
- For a 10-minute mile, add 14 calories to the base number.
- For a 25-minute mile, subtract 7 calories from the base number.

How far will you have to go to lose a pound of fat? A pound of fat contains 3,500 calories. Take your base number you arrived at above and divide it into 3,500. To lose a pound of fat, our 150-lb. person will have to walk about 46 miles. That's enough walking to rival Forrest Gump, which is why successful weight loss programs insist on losing no more than one to two pounds a week.

Look at a map of your community to design a route that will suit your needs. Consider distance and terrain. Remember to warm up with about 10 minutes of stretching.

- Lift one heel to your rear and grab your ankle. Hold for a few seconds, then, leaning on a chair or wall for support, lift your ankle up to stretch your upper thigh (quadriceps). Repeat with other leg.
- Press your toes against a wall and straighten your leg to stretch your calf. This also works well to loosen cramped muscles.
- You'll be using your upper body on a brisk walk, so don't forget to stretch here too. Take your right arm over your head and touch your left shoulder. Grab your right elbow to pull gently on your arm. Then pull the same arm across your body to feel the stretch in your upper back and shoulder. Repeat on the other side.

Don't just flop into an easy chair after an hour of intensive walking. Gradually slow down your pace to allow your body a chance to recover.

While walking is fairly easy on your body, if you have a heart condition, asthma or any other ailment that you think might make walking risky, check with your doctor. And listen to your body—if your muscles are sore, give them a rest for a day or two.

HOW MANY CALORIES DO YOU BURN?

Type of Activity	Calories used/hour	Examples
Sedentary	80 to 110	Eating, office work, reading, sewing, typing, writing and watching television
Light	150 to 240	Dancing slowly, ironing and riding power lawn mower
Moderate	240 to 300	Bowling, cleaning windows, cycling slowly, fishing, food shopping, light gardening, mopping floors, pushing light power mower, vacuuming and walking at moderate pace
	300 to 360	Badminton, calisthenics, cycling at moderate pace, scrubbing floors, table tennis, doubles tennis and walking faster than normal
Vigorous	360 to 420	Fast cycling, ice skating, roller skating, in-line skating and walking briskly
	420 to 480	Dancing fast, horseback trotting, pushing hand mower, singles tennis and water skiing
	480 to 600	Basketball, downhill skiing, horseback galloping, jogging slowly, sawing hard wood and speed cycling
Strenuous	600 to 660	Running 5.5 mph and swimming breast stroke
	More than 660	Handball, running faster than 6.6 mph, cross-country skiing, squash

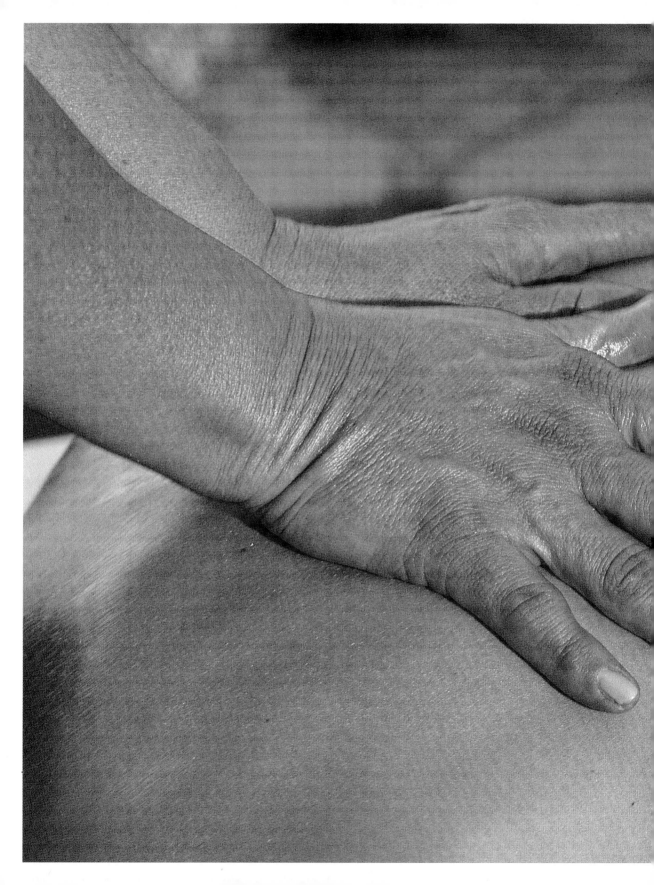

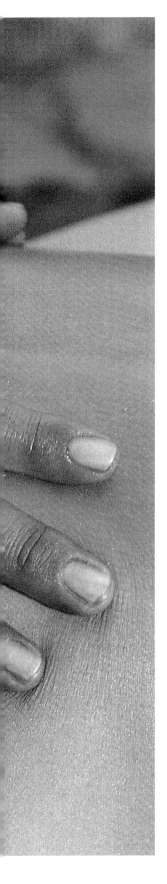

Healing Hands

Say the word *spa*, and the image inevitably comes to mind of towelled people lying prone on tables while burly masseuses with names like Helga and Sven karate chop their backs. Most massage is of the Swedish variety, but many spas offer different variations on that theme, including the ancient arts of shiatsu and reiki, and treatments that involve finding and activating certain pressure points, such as reflexology.

SORE MUSCLES?

Everyone gets a stiff back or tight shoulder occasionally. Unfortunately, for some people, chronic pain is the norm. There are many causes of chronic muscle pain, such as arthritis, rheumatism, fibromyalgia and chronic fatigue syndrome, which may be difficult to prevent. The good news is that a lot of muscle pain can be avoided. It is mostly caused by repetitive strain, and breaking the cycle can do wonders.

- If your job involves sitting or standing in the same position all day, take mini exercise breaks to stimulate circulation. Even walking on the spot for a few minutes helps.
- Set a watch or clock alarm to remind you to do hourly posture checks. Chances are your shoulders are hunched around your ears as you lean toward the computer screen, or you're slouching in your chair as you go over those reports.
- If you carry a heavy bag, alternate sides, or better yet, switch to a backpack, which distributes weight more evenly on your back. Switch arms when carrying a child.
- Your computer screen should be eye-level. Having it positioned too high or too low could cause neck strain. If your chair offers no lower-back support, a small pillow or rolled-up towel will help.
- Above all, listen to your body. If it hurts, give it a rest. Although that may be impractical, you can at least attempt to alter the way you lift, type, drive or whatever.

WHAT MAKES YOUR MUSCLES TENSE

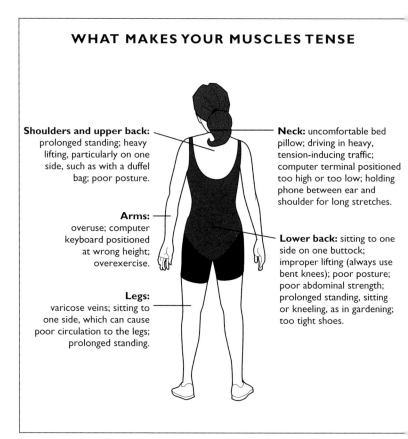

Shoulders and upper back: prolonged standing; heavy lifting, particularly on one side, such as with a duffel bag; poor posture.

Neck: uncomfortable bed pillow; driving in heavy, tension-inducing traffic; computer terminal positioned too high or too low; holding phone between ear and shoulder for long stretches.

Arms: overuse; computer keyboard positioned at wrong height; overexercise.

Lower back: sitting to one side on one buttock; improper lifting (always use bent knees); poor posture; poor abdominal strength; prolonged standing, sitting or kneeling, as in gardening; too tight shoes.

Legs: varicose veins; sitting to one side, which can cause poor circulation to the legs; prolonged standing.

It isn't just a luxurious way to spend an afternoon; massage therapy is a legitimate alternative to pain- and stress-relieving drugs, which can become expensive, not to mention addictive. A massage stimulates the circulatory and lymphatic systems, helping to prevent water retention and slowing down the formation of cellulite. It also helps you eliminate metabolic wastes more quickly, making more room for more oxygen and nutrients to reach cells and tissues.

Your body is a repository for emotional, physical and psychological pain. The feeling of someone's touch wakes up your skin, and your muscles let go of long-held tension, getting your energy flowing more freely. This often leads to deeper, more relaxing breathing and sometimes provides relief from tension headaches and eye strains. The reduced stress can allow you to think more clearly and express yourself emotionally.

Massage therapy developed from our animal instinct to want to be touched. It's no wonder that the simple act of holding an ill person's hand can promote healing. Unfortunately, sexual taboos in this part of the world have made touching and being touched awkward for some people. If you've had a professional massage before, you may remember being slightly on edge when hands came close to a sensitive area such as the lower back, also known as the upper buttocks. It may take a few minutes to get into the groove, but eventually you'll relax and enjoy the feeling of a massage. There's also a psychological benefit to massage therapy. For some, it's the act of taking a break that is rejuvenating; for others it's a boost for their self-esteem to say, "Hey, I'm worth it."

If your job requires you to stay in the same position for hours on end, such as on an assembly line, in a car or at a computer, you're probably a prime candidate for regular massage therapy.

Solo Massage

There are a number of techniques you can use to loosen up stiff muscles by yourself. To start, warm up your skin. Moisten your hands with a lubricant of your choice, preferably a non-petroleum product. Starting at your heel, move flat hands in semi-circles one at a time up the calf. This is known as effleurage. Continue all the way up your leg to your buttock. For the top part of thighs, push the skin away from you with the butt of your hand, alternating hands in semi-circular motion. Keep adding lotion or massage oil as needed.

To warm up hard-to-reach places such as back and neck, you may want to try a heating pad or hot water bottle. (A shower or hot bath is also an excellent tonic for stiff muscles.)

There are a number of manufactured self-massagers on the market today, ranging from wooden-handled rollers to electronic "yokes" that prod and poke worn neck muscles. You can find samples in novelty stores or up-scale gift shops. Or try your kitchen cupboard. A rolling pin or a can of soup has a similar effect at a much cheaper cost. Once your muscles are warm and ready to be plied (about 15 minutes of friction rubbing), you can get started.

REIKI

Japanese for "universal life energy," reiki employs a light hand touch to transfer a flow of energy from the massager to the massagee. Proponents of reiki believe it creates balance, harmony and well-being.

WHEN NOT TO GET A MASSAGE

If you have any of these conditions, check with your doctor to see if massage is safe for you:

- varicose veins
- heart problems
- skin conditions such as psoriasis
- inflammatory diseases such as arthritis
- lymphatic or skin cancer
- infectious diseases
- inflamed or infected injuries
- areas of heavy tissue damage
- recent broken bones
- high blood pressure

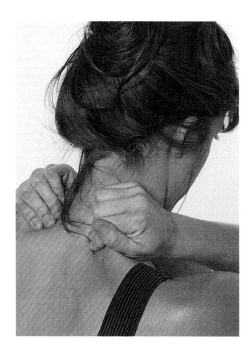

Using your fingers or a commercial massager, rub the sides of your neck avoiding the vertebrae.

SHIATSU

Based on the 2,000-year-old Chinese art of acupuncture, a shiatsu (or acupressure) massage stimulates certain pressure points on the body. Advocates of shiatsu believe life energy flows through the body in 14 different channels, or meridians. Each meridian is connected to different organs, and by tapping into these meridians at specific points, the organ can be energized and hopefully be made to feel better. The goal is to balance the two opposite flows of energy in the body, known as the yin and yang.

Legs: Sit with feet elevated on the sofa or a footstool so that your muscles feel flaccid. Start by pushing your calf muscle from your knee to your heel. Use a flat hand, fingers together. For the thighs, take a rolling pin or can of soup and "roll" the muscles on your upper thigh.

Arms: Here's where the soup cans comes in again. Holding it in one hand, rub it up and down along your upper arm, then your lower arm. You can also rub your forearm with your hand. With fingers together on one side, and thumb on the other side, gently push and pull the skin on your arm.

Back and Neck: Without the benefit of a manufactured massager, this area is pretty tricky to reach. However, some yoga stretches can produce the same effect. First, take the tie from a bathrobe, a necktie or even a piece of rope. Wrap the ends of the tie around your hands a couple of times until the length is such that you look like the letter Y with arms outstretched. Drop your left arm and bend it up toward the center of your back. Raise your right arm, but drop your hand toward the center of your back. By gently pulling the tie up and down, you are massaging the muscles along your spine.

For the neck, drape the tie around the back of your head and tuck your chin forward. Don't pull on the tie, but allow the weight of your arms to stretch out the back of your neck. Stretch the muscles on the side of your neck in the same way, leaning your head to one side, gently weighting the tie with your hands.

Partner Massage

Definitely the way to go, massaging or being massaged by a partner can be a real treat. The toughest part is determining who goes first, so have a coin ready for flipping.

In the likely event you don't own a massage table, arrange some pillows on the floor. The hard surface is more ideal than a spongy bed—a futon is a great compromise. The first to be massaged lies down on his or her front, arms relaxed at sides (not over the head, which tenses neck and shoulder muscles) with face down, if possible,

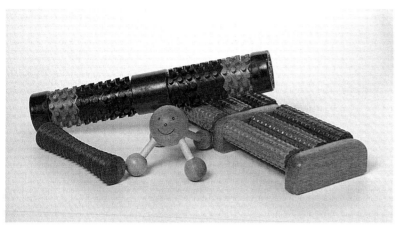

TOP: Solo massage can be enhanced with manufactured massagers like these, which make it easier to work hard-to-reach places.

BOTTOM: Gently pushing or pulling on the skin of the forearm helps relieve stiff muscles.

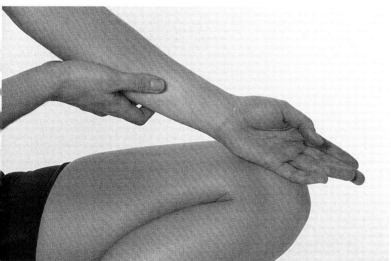

to avoid neck strain. If you can't find a comfortable arrangement with pillows supporting your head, turn your head to the side. (At a spa, you would be naked with a sheet tucked around your hips and legs. If you're not comfortable with the idea of stripping down for someone, wear a tank top and a pair of loose-fitting shorts.) As in the solo massage, start with some oil and friction rubbing to heat up the skin.

Back: Using flat palms, stroke the back from shoulder to waist, moving from one side to the other. Once the skin feels warm to the touch, slide your thumb and palm along either side of the spine, taking care to avoid vertebrae. Push the folds of skin up with fingertips, moving

HYDROTHERAPY

In a sense, hydrotherapy is at the heart of all natural spas—using water as a curative element. Everyone knows a nice warm bath relieves sore muscles, relaxes and rejuvenates the skin. Hydrotherapy takes it a step further and alternates between hot and cold water to stimulate blood circulation.

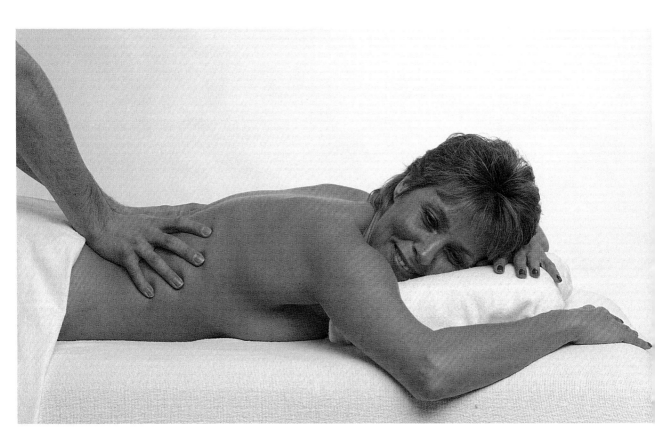

Line the massage surface with a towel and, if the massagee finds it uncomfortable to lie face down, provide a pillow.

all the way down to the lower back. Don't forget—the back ends at the tailbone, not at the waist, so you must massage the upper buttocks for a complete workover.

Legs: Starting at the top of the legs, "walk" your hands in a C-shape (as if you're holding a cup) toward the foot, scooping the muscle as you go.

Shoulders: To access the shoulder blade, gently move the arm so the back of your partner's hand is touching the small of his or her back. Using both thumbs, press along the muscle lining the blade, holding each point for about 15 seconds. Then, placing both hands on one shoulder, pull the muscle from front to back, one hand after the other. Use mainly the palms of your hands and work from the neck out. Repeat on other side.

Arms: Standing beside your partner and facing the same way, use the same C-scooping motion you used on the legs, starting at the shoulder and working to the elbow. Then move so your left hip is at the massagee's right hip and take the same arm in both hands. Holding the arm at the elbow, pull the skin of the forearm on one side with the right hand, then the other side with the left hand. Repeat this pulling motion several times.

Hands: Finish the arm by gently massaging the hand (turn the fingers up so you can use your thumb on the palm). Move into the muscular part between the thumb and forefinger and gently pinch. Use your thumb and forefinger to rub and pull each finger from hand to tip. When you've finished, test to see how relaxed your partner is—if the arm is loose and floppy, you're on the right track. Gently replace arm at your partner's side.

Neck: Holding the towel up in front of you, ask your partner to roll over and cover him or herself. Most armchair massage enthusiasts miss this key position in giving a friend a back rub. It allows the neck muscles to "hang," thereby allowing you to work them that much more thoroughly. Standing at your partner's head, slip your hands beneath both shoulders and place them on the upper spine. Slide your hands along the spine, continuing along the neck and resting at the head. Hold the head up with your thumbs behind the ears and your fingers under the base of the skull. The weight of your partner's head against your fingertips activates a natural pressure point along the top of the neck.

Face: The face is often neglected in body massages, but it shouldn't be. From daily tension to headaches to eye strain—we harbor it all in the muscles of our face. Place fingertips or knuckles above the center of the eyes at the hairline. Massage in tiny circles, working down to the middle of the forehead.

Next, place knuckles or fingertips on the bones under the ends of the eyebrows next to the nose. Move fingers in a circular motion along the brow bone, resting at the outer edge of the eyes.

Scalp: The simplest way to soothe and massage the scalp is to pretend you're washing your partner's hair. Run your fingers through the hair, section by section, gently tugging on the ends to release tension in the scalp.

For an extra-soothing finish to a body massage, try this Asian technique: Soak a towel in hot water and wring it out. Lay it over the massagee's back to help the massage oil penetrate. If towel seems too hot, spin it in the air a few times to make the temperature more accommodating.

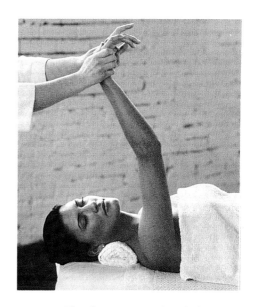

For a good hand massage, gently rub the muscular area between the thumb and forefinger.

Don't forget to ply the massagee's scalp! Pretend you're washing your partner's hair.

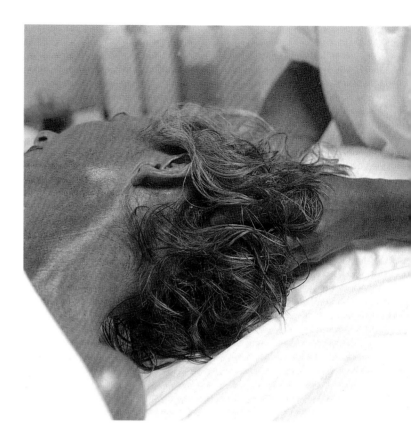

Chest: The chest is an extension of the neck and shoulders and is an area that should not be missed, although it's a sensitive area because it approaches some erogenous zones. Still standing at the head of your partner, place your hands just below the chin. Using the palm and butt of your hands to gently push away the skin, work from one side to the other.

Legs: Moving to your partner's hip, facing his or her feet, place both hands on the upper thigh. With C-shaped hands, push skin toward knee, alternating hands.

Feet: Extend the leg massage to the feet, pressing thumbs in a semi-circular motion on the soles of the feet. Stand with your back to your partner's head, and pull the foot toward you. With your fingers on the top of the foot and your thumbs on the sole, concentrate on pressure points such as the heel and the ball of the foot. Knead the instep

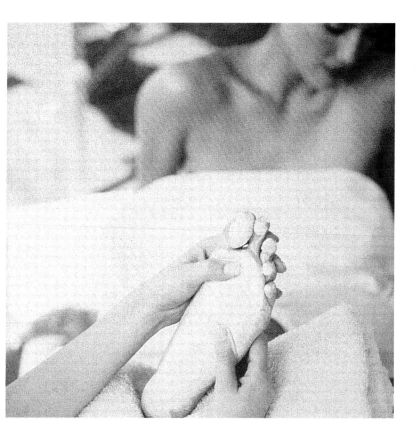

Pent-up stress can take its toll on your tootsies, so remember to include your feet at the end of a body massage.

of the foot with your knuckles. Finish by squeezing and lightly tugging on each toe. Repeat on other foot.

Note: Although not every square inch of the body has muscle to massage, lightly rubbing with lubricated hands is still a great way to relieve tension.

Massage for Hire

If you're looking to really splurge, hiring a registered massage therapist (RMT) to come to your home is truly the way to be good to yourself. RMTs are highly trained in anatomical and physiological workings and have the added benefit of being able to assess the cause of your body's weak spots. An RMT should ask for a confidential medical history and may be able to suggest exercises that will help

Reward yourself! Choose a non-calorie reward like a massage or a facial every time you fulfill your weekly workout goals.

—*Sheila Cluff, The Oaks and The Palms, California*

prevent tension from creeping back so quickly. Though it may seem somewhat disconcerting at first to be so exposed to a complete stranger, a massage therapist working in your home or at his or her office is a professional. However, if you do feel the slightest bit uncomfortable, an RMT should work in whatever condition suits you provided he or she can perform an adequate massage. On the first session, and possibly subsequent ones, RMTs should tell you what they are going to do every step of the way and why. They will also ask you if their touch is too hard or too soft. Some like to talk, some keep quiet; usually they just follow your lead. Many massage therapists also like to scent the room, turn the lights low and play quiet music to help you relax.

After the massage is over, the RMT will leave the room and give you time to ease back into the real world or, in some cases, wake up. Take your time here. Even the busiest massage centers allow for this recuperative time, for both the client and the RMT, who needs to rest his or her body before starting with the next lucky customer. Sit up gradually and take a few deep breaths to supercharge your muscles with oxygen. Get dressed slowly and try to keep that relaxed feeling as long as you can.

For information about how to find a massage therapist, contact your provincial or state association, or try a spa, salon or fitness club near you. They may rent out employees or be able to recommend someone.

REFLEXOLOGY Reflexology, like shiatsu (acupressure), is based on the principle that your body is lined with 14 meridians, each connected to different organs and bodily functions. The meridians end in your hands and feet, and by pressing certain trigger points, you can alleviate symptoms elsewhere in your body. (See diagram of foot on page 72.) A reflexologist can often tell if you're having digestive problems, for example, by feeling the tension in the corresponding part of the foot. Some massage therapists practice reflexology exclusively; others include elements of the ancient therapy in more traditional massages. However, more and more spas are offering reflexology massages, particularly recommending them as a prelude to manicures

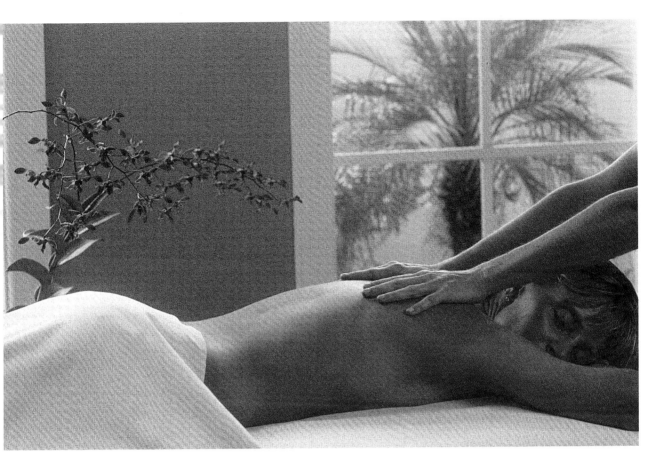

and pedicures. The advantage of reflexology is that you can perform it on yourself just as easily as a friend can.

Hands: As in all massage, the hand must be warm and lubricated. Work your favorite moisturizer into your skin. Start the massage by squeezing the fleshy, muscled part of the hand between the thumb and first finger, with your thumb on the top side. This brings relief for headaches and is also good for constipation or other colon problems. Massage the entire palm area with the thumb. Starting from the outside, work in a circular motion to the inside. Apply pressure points around the circle, holding each for at least 30 seconds. If the spot is particularly tender, hold for two to three minutes until you feel tension bubble away. Massage each finger and thumb, accessing pressure points.

Having a registered massage therapist come to you is the ultimate in pampering.

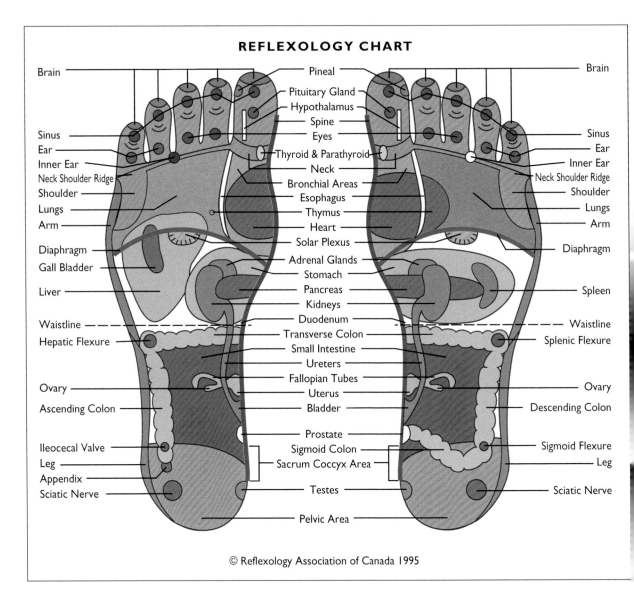

REFLEXOLOGY CHART

Brain — Pineal — Brain
Pituitary Gland
Hypothalamus
Spine
Sinus — Eyes — Sinus
Ear — Ear
Inner Ear — Thyroid & Parathyroid — Inner Ear
Neck Shoulder Ridge — Neck — Neck Shoulder Ridge
Shoulder — Bronchial Areas — Shoulder
Esophagus
Lungs — Thymus — Lungs
Arm — Heart — Arm
Solar Plexus
Diaphragm — Diaphragm
Gall Bladder — Adrenal Glands
Stomach
Liver — Pancreas — Spleen
Kidneys
Duodenum
Waistline — — — Transverse Colon — — — Waistline
Hepatic Flexure — Small Intestine — Splenic Flexure
Ureters
Fallopian Tubes
Ovary — Uterus — Ovary
Ascending Colon — Bladder — Descending Colon
Prostate
Ileocecal Valve — Sigmoid Colon — Sigmoid Flexure
Leg — Sacrum Coccyx Area — Leg
Appendix
Sciatic Nerve — Testes — Sciatic Nerve
Pelvic Area

© Reflexology Association of Canada 1995

Feet: After soaking feet in warm water and softening calluses, start by locating the inverted Y that runs from the center of the foot to either side of the heel. Press along the Y with your thumb to relieve stress. For overall muscle cramping and tension, massage the lower calf (this is easier to do on someone else than on yourself). Holding the foot, run flat palms from the top of the toes up calf to knee. How much pressure to apply is up to the individual—use your partner as a gauge. Then stroke the calf, one hand following the other, down to the heel and toe. Massage up the calf, moving thumb pads in a half-moon upward stroke (known as petrissage, a useful technique in any kind of massage). Come down either side of the calf, making little circles stopping at the top part of the foot. Rub your thumb along the foot away from the toes to the top and outside of the ankle. Massaging back along the top of the foot, move to the bottom of the foot using the petrissage motion. Start at the heel, move along to the flat part and stop at the toes.

For the toes, which correspond to the head and sinuses, move each in little circles to the left and right. Gently massage each toe, finishing off with a tug. Make circles with your thumb on the heel, wrapping other fingers around top of the foot. Stroke the flat part of the foot with your thumbs.

To effectively activate the pressure points on the bottom of your foot by yourself, try rolling your foot on a golf ball or tennis ball.

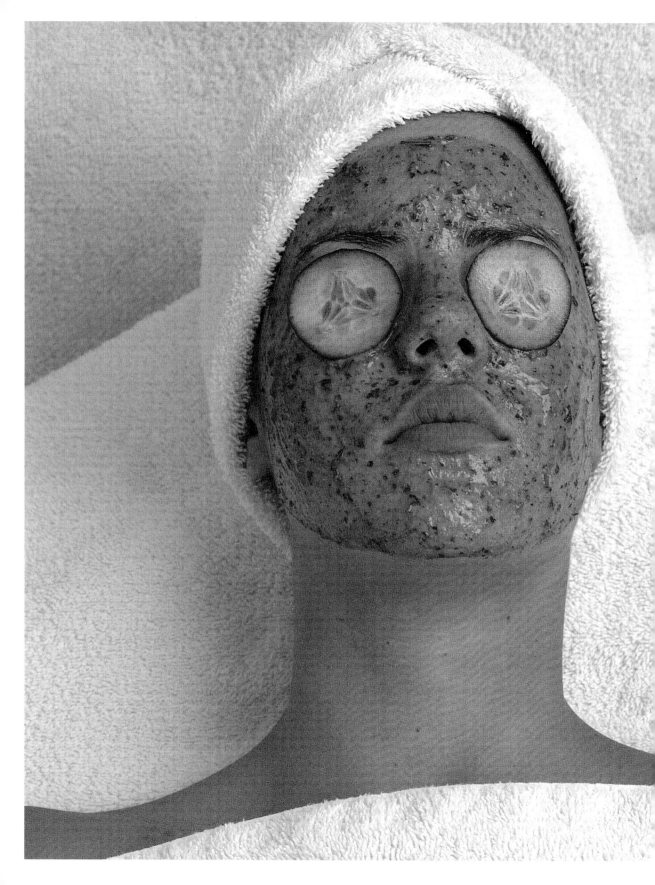

Body and Beauty Treatments

Before you renounce as the stuff of hedonism a long soak in a warm, fragrant tub with your body slathered in apricot facial scrub, think again. Sure, these spa treatments are pure pleasure, but make no mistake—they're also good for you. Your skin and hair need therapy just as your tired muscles need a massage. And neglecting problem skin or unhealthy hair has a twofold effect—not only does your appearance sag, but your spirits slump right along with it. You can scour the salons and drugstores for your favorite products, or try some of our homemade recipes.

Skin Basics

Whoever said beauty is only skin deep had it right. While clear, healthy skin may not get noticed immediately, uneven, blemished skin usually greets people before you do. Today's arsenal of make-up products makes it so easy to cover up skin problems with (aptly named) "cover-up" that getting and maintaining healthy skin often falls by the wayside.

If you start to take the steps outlined in Chapter 3 to improve your health, don't be surprised if clearer skin is a positive side effect. If your skin is dry, oily or both, and changing diet and activity levels seems to have no effect, don't despair. There are other factors at work. First, a lesson in biology.

Skin is made up of three main layers.

- Epidermis (the top layer), which is further divided into the corneal layer (dead skin on the very outside) and living cells that are preparing to replace the corneal layer as it dies off. This is the strongest layer of skin, though not the thickest, because it forms a protective barrier between the rest of your body and the elements.
- Dermis (the middle layer), a mesh of collagen and tissue, supports sebaceous glands (which secrete natural oils), hair follicles and their muscles, and sweat glands. The natural oils, or sebum, combine with lipids to form a protective barrier on the surface of the skin. Sweat glands maintain the skin's pH balance and help flush dirt and oil from the pores.
- Subcutis (the bottom layer), which is basically underlying fat tissue.

Your skin is constantly manufacturing fresh cells in the epidermis layer. It takes about 28 days for keratinocytes (living skin cells) to work their way from the bottom of the epidermis to the outside world. The cycle perhaps explains why some women find acne break-outs or skin sensitivity coincides with their menstrual periods.

The epidermis also churns out melanocytes, which produce melanin, our bodies' built-in sunscreen. When our skin is exposed to burning ultraviolet rays, melanin protects skin cells by darkening them. If you spend years worshipping the sun, your body's second line of defense kicks in—skin thickening, resulting in a brown, leathery appearance.

Oily Skin

Oily skin is the result of overactive sebaceous glands, a trait that is often inherited or provoked in warm, humid weather. Oil production can also reach geyser proportions when your body is under stress or trauma. Oily skin is most commonly found on the dreaded T-zone—the forehead, nose and chin—but is not restricted to that area. Don't make the mistake of bombarding oily skin with harsh toners or astringents. They will dry your skin, then trigger your sebaceous glands to overcompensate by producing more oil. Instead, look for water-based moisturizers (they'll usually use words like "hydra" and "hydrating" on the label) that will keep the skin moist and slow oil production.

Dry Skin

Dry skin is less a function of heredity and more a function of environment and aging. Most women over 55 have dry skin, as depleting hormones slow production in the sebaceous glands. Harmful ultraviolet light from the sun, air pollution and hermetically sealed, dry office buildings also play a major role in sapping the skin of its ability to stay comfortably moist. Skin draws water from its perennially moist living epidermal and dermal layers, then retains that moisture by regulating how fast it moves through the corneal layer. In dry skin, the transport of water is very rapid. Without an adequate supply of water in the corneal layer, the protective barrier cannot function properly. The solution, oddly enough, is the same remedy as for oily skin—keep your dermis hydrated in order to keep skin composition balanced. Moisturizers designed for dry skin typically feel richer to the touch.

How to Define Your Skin Type

Most people have a good idea what's wrong with their skin. After all, you've been living with it all your life. A simple way to check is to

DO YOU HAVE DIMPLES WHERE YOU DON'T WANT THEM?

Cellulite creams have been crowding the infomercial market of late, but don't be fooled. Those little divots in your thighs and buttocks can't be cured with a simple potion.

Believed by some to be a form of water retention (unique to women), cellulite is encouraged by a sedentary lifestyle and lack of exercise. Some doctors theorize that toxins circulating in the bloodstream— such as alcohol, nicotine, pollution, saturated fat, food additives and chemicals—clog fat cells. The capillaries dilate and eventually the lymphatic system is too overworked to drain the excess fluid away. The area then gets a case of the jiggles.

You can give cellulite the bum's rush by (a) watching toxin intake, (b) getting more exercise and (c) stimulating the lymphatic system by brushing and massaging the skin. Cypress, geranium and rosemary, used in aromatherapy massage, have all been found to help discourage cellulite formation.

Cellulite creams or treatments may not be a complete washout, however, because they have to be rubbed in thoroughly, which helps stimulate the lymphatic system. (Some may also contain the above active ingredients.) But you'll probably get similar results using a soft-bristle body brush and your favorite moisturizer, combined with decreased toxin exposure and a stepped-up exercise program.

Mud and other types of facial masks draw out impurities as they dry on the skin.

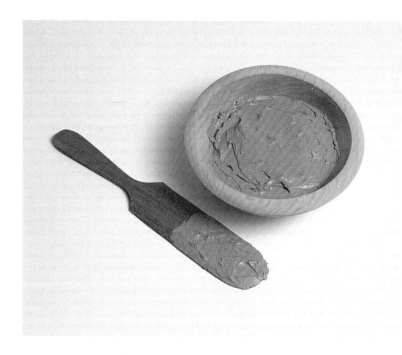

look in the mirror—shiny skin usually denotes oily skin, and flaky skin usually points to dry skin. But that's just a superficial analysis. Blackheads—pores clogged with oils and dirt—could be lurking beyond the surface of the seemingly clearest skin, invisible to the naked eye. The best way to find out is to visit an esthetician for skin analysis and a facial.

BUYER BEWARE

If some cosmetics did what they actually claim they do, they'd have to go through the rigors of federal drug testing. Few do, so be skeptical of outlandish marketing claims that promise to reverse the hands of time. These products aren't going to be harmful, but they likely won't have the hoped-for end result. And for the bucks, why take the risk?

What a Facial Does for You

A facial, like so many spa treatments, enhances both body and soul. Aside from the initial shock of putting your skin under the microscope—okay, a giant magnifying glass—the gentle massage and cooling masks of a professional facial are a great stress reliever. Not surprisingly, estheticians recommend monthly facials to prevent bouts of acne or severe dry skin, known as eczema. Indeed, in some European countries, facialists require nursing and medical backgrounds.

A thorough facial follows six basic steps: skin analysis; steaming and deep cleaning (professionals sometimes use mini-vacuums or extraction tools to dig out blackheads and whiteheads); massage; at least one mask specially selected, and in some cases, concocted, for your skin's specific needs; mask removal; moisturizer application.

People with severe acne or overly sensitive skin should avoid the steam treatment—it tends to aggravate the condition by bringing all the blood to the surface. Many professionals also eschew the high-tech gizmos in the deep-cleaning phase, favoring the old-fashioned but efficient massage method.

While skin analysis and blackhead extraction might require a more practiced eye or hand, there's nothing to stop you from adopting the other components of a professional facial in your health and beauty routine.

Masks, which draw out dirt, oil and other impurities as they dry on the skin, can be used once a week for hydrating and toning skin. Choose one formulated especially for your skin type. Some spas suggest masks with only natural ingredients. Chamomile and aloe vera prevent skin from becoming red and blotchy; avocado and banana-based masks are good for dry skin, while strawberry and cucumber absorb excess sebum in oily skin. Clay-based masks (or, in some cases, a plastering of pure mud) also absorb oils, and the tiny grains of earth help exfoliate and buff the skin. People with dry skin may find masks with natural exfoliants such as oatmeal or apricot seeds more satisfying. The mild abrasives help slough off the dead skin cells on the surface.

Follow recipes or read manufacturers' directions carefully—many warn against applying the mask to the delicate eye area. Most require five to fifteen minutes to "set," during which time you should relax, not talk, and keep your face immobile. Some masks are formulated to harden into a gel to be peeled off, others should dry out until they're ready to be rubbed off.

The final moisturizing phase is necessary to protect your face. Remember, you've just essentially scrubbed off the top layer of dead skin and exposed a new layer. That skin is extra-vulnerable, so be sure to apply a sunscreen with a minimum SPF of 15. A good facial can act almost like a mini-facelift. And think of the money you'll save!

OPEN UP

For decades the cosmetic industry has had people thinking one product will open pores and the next will close them. Don't believe it. Our pores do no such thing. However, it is important to clean out pores as dirt, make-up and oil can plug them up. Hot water or steam helps soften pores, enabling the dirt to come away more readily. After your skin has been cleaned, pores tend to look smaller, hence the image of opening and closing. And smaller pores give the skin a smoother and more porcelain-like look.

Unfortunately, pores can't be sealed off from the outside world like little manholes. Regular cleaning with a mild cleanser or astringent is enough to keep pores unnoticed and functioning properly.

OPPOSITE: Moisturizers are a key ingredient in any facial—at home or in a spa. Always finish off your treatment by replacing the moisture the skin has lost.

Natural Facials and Other Popular Spa Treatments

Basic Facial

First, cover your hair with a shower cap or a towel to get it out of the way. After removing all traces of make-up, mix cornmeal or oatmeal with a little moisturizer or water; alternatively, use beauty grains, available at most cosmetic counters. Massage the paste gently into your face, avoiding areas with broken capillaries (tiny blood vessels). This light exfoliation gets rid of old skin cells as well as stimulating collagen production deep in the skin's dermis. Rinse well and pat dry.

Next, dip cotton make-up remover pads in cold herbal tea and place them over the eyes. Lie back and leave the pads on for a few minutes to reduce puffiness. Apply eye cream or a dab of honey under the eyes to lighten dark circles.

To the rest of your face, apply a commercial mask for your skin type, or use lemon juice mixed with either plain yogurt or beaten egg whites. Recline with this mixture on for about 15 minutes (or as package directs). Rinse well. Finally, apply your favorite moisturizer to damp skin.

Moisturizing Facial

Fill a bowl with boiling water and add a chamomile tea bag. Lean over the bowl and cover your head with a towel to form a tent over the bowl. Ensure your face is about 10 inches from the bowl and wait five to eight minutes.

Using a cleansing milk, gently massage your face, moving fingers in small circular patterns from the throat to the chin and then chin to jaw line and over the cheeks in upward motions. Massage in circles around the eyes, moving inward to the nose, then from the center of the forehead outward.

Splash face with lukewarm water and pat dry.

FOR DRY SKIN Use a hydrating mask loaded with natural moisturizers. Mix half and half (a few tablespoons each) crushed avocado and papaya with one tablespoon of honey.

FOR OILY SKIN Use a clay-based mask to soak up excess facial oils and draw out impurities. Blend a tablespoon each of olive oil, honey and moisturizer with a puréed lemon and a few drops of Vitamins E and A and an egg yolk.

Apply either mask over face and neck, avoiding eyes. After 15 to 20 minutes, use lukewarm water to remove the mask, and spritz your face with mineral water. Blot dry and apply moisturizer.

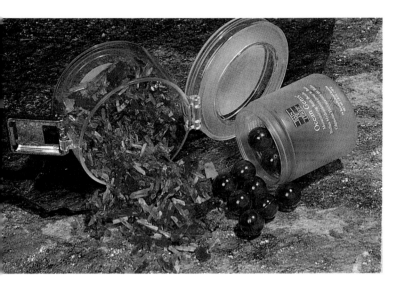

Wrinkle Remover

Beaten egg whites are a miracle mix when it comes to disguising wrinkles for a few hours. Using a small pointed paintbrush, simply fill in small lines with the egg-white mixture. Let dry before carefully applying make-up.

Using the egg-white mixture as a mask also helps disguise wrinkles, and the protein in the eggs is good for your skin. Apply mixture to face and neck. Allow to harden for 10 to 15 minutes. Rinse off with warm water and pat dry.

Soothing Face Fix

Mash one ripe avocado and spread it all over your face. Leave on for 20 minutes, then rinse. The natural oil from the avocado moisturizes and rejuvenates those overexposed facial skin cells.

SURGICAL SOLUTIONS

For some people, plastic surgery is the solution to feeling better about themselves. Personal appearance is so tightly linked to emotional health that pronounced skin changes can be a devastating blow to the ego. The following are services that should be performed by a medical doctor only. Plastic surgeons, dermatologists, even some family physicians offer these treatments. Verify your specialist's credentials and insist on patient references.

Dermabrasion—Commonly used to treat acne scarring. Top layer of skin is carefully sanded down to the pink. Patients must keep new skin well lubricated for weeks while new skin cells form.

Laser surgery—Used to treat acne scarring and remove tiny wrinkles. Local anesthetic used while CO_2 laser literally burns skin, to the degree of a severe sunburn. Laser has more accuracy than dermabrasion, and recovery is much quicker and less painful.

Collagen injections—Collagen—fat molecules derived from cow proteins—is injected under the surface of the skin to fill in tiny lines or to enhance fullness of lips or chin, for example. Temporary treatment that must be repeated every six months or so after body has absorbed and eliminated collagen.

ANTI-WRINKLE STRATEGIES

Until recent cosmetic innovations, the only thing that could prevent wrinkles was staying out of the sun. Pale faces were once hailed as paragons of beauty. Around the middle of this century, however, tanned faces were deemed healthier and more appealing. But those who as teens slathered on the baby oil and lay out with reflector screens are now paying the price with skin that has aged before its time. Of course, with the realization that too much sun at an early age can lead to skin cancer, the pendulum is swinging back. Paler, smoother skin is returning into vogue. Dermatologists recommend everyone should wear at least 15 SPF sunscreen at all times outdoors. A moisturizer that includes sunscreen is ideal.

However, there is some hope for small wrinkles, the kind that appear only when your face is animated. (Permanent wrinkles under the chin or in the forehead, for example, can be done away with only by cosmetic surgery, which is about as far away from the spa experience as you can get.) Alpha hydroxy acids (known as AHAs) are found in many spa products and come from three naturally occurring sources: glycolic acid, derived from sugar cane; citric acid, derived from citrus fruits; and lactic acid, derived from milk.

AHAs have actually been around for ages. Legend has it that Cleopatra, who was noted for her excellent skin and attention to beauty, used to bathe in sour milk. Today's products containing AHAs vary in effectiveness according to the percentage of AHA contained.

AHAs work by gently exfoliating the top layer of skin. The natural acid makes it more penetrating than, say, a simple scrub with a loofah. AHAs smooth rough, dry areas and refine uneven, textured skin. They also help fade age spots or other skin pigmentations (including freckles!). Because the skin is losing a layer, wrinkles appear less noticeable because they aren't quite as deep.

Sensitive skins may find AHAs to be too harsh. It's a good idea to test a patch of skin on the underside of your forearm (wait a couple of days for a delayed reaction) before treating your entire face.

Many spas offer AHA peels. Several cosmetics, including foundation, moisturizer and even lipstick, are now available with AHAs. Most commercial products limit AHAs to 8% strength, but there is no labeling legislation in place to ensure the consumer knows what she's buying. AHA content that's not much higher than 8% can do damage to the skin's natural protective barrier. Dermatologists, for example, use AHAs at 15% to 40% concentration when doing acid peels.

Renova is the latest wrinkle fighter to join in the anti-aging crusade. In 1995 the Federal Drug Administration in the United States approved tretinoin (known by its product name as Renova) as a treatment for wrinkles. Health Canada soon followed suit.

In testing creams containing tretinoin, researchers found the drug appears to reduce fine facial wrinkles, fade age spots, stimulate collagen production and prolong the life of the top layer of skin cells, which are shed prematurely due to sun exposure. There is even some evidence that tretinoin may prevent sun damage. However, there are side effects: temporary peeling, redness, blistering and a permanent increase in sun sensitivity. Renova is available through prescription only.

Body Wraps and Exfoliation

Facials address the need to exfoliate dead skin cells on the face. But just because other parts of your body may be under wrap, don't ignore them. Exfoliating everywhere is an important step toward healthier, smoother skin.

Daily bathing usually gets rid of a lot of the dead cells; so does shaving (that's why men seem to age more slowly than women—constant facial exfoliation). But if you use a natural sea sponge or a loofah to scrub your skin, you'll do a more thorough job.

Not only is exfoliating good for your skin, it also feels pretty nice. If your shower is fitted with a fancy shower head, here's your chance to use the different settings. Even if your shower head is army issue, let the water beat down on tense body parts, such as neck, shoulders and lower back. If the head is attached to a hose, take advantage of it and spray the soles of your feet.

The basic rules of exfoliating are (1) use a mild abrasive, such as a loofah combined with a grainy paste and (2) replace the moisture you took away with a good moisturizer. Try these homemade solutions.

Loofah Body Polish

- Start a hot shower running to let the bathroom get good and steamy, while you mix two cups of mineral salts, sea salts (fine) or Epsom salts (available in health, drug and grocery stores), with one-half cup of avocado oil, olive oil or light body lotion to make a thin paste.
- Standing in the shower, apply a handful of paste to your skin, starting at the feet. Work the paste in a circular motion, up the legs, over the buttocks, stomach, arms and chest, paying special attention to rough spots on knees, elbows and heels. (Do not use on face or other sensitive areas.)
- Rinse off in warm shower and pat dry.
- Apply your favorite body lotion or avocado lotion to seal in moisture and protect the skin.

Herbal Wrap

Herbal wraps detoxify the body by causing you to sweat out impurities. Some spas continue the wrap for an hour, but that's too debilitating when doing it on your own. Try 20 minutes.

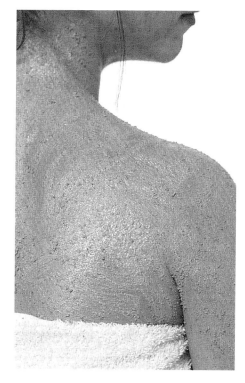

A grainy paste applied to your body is an excellent exfoliant. Scrub gently with a sea sponge or loofah and rinse.

Loofahs and natural sponges give exfoliating a little boost, and help you slough off dead skin more effectively.

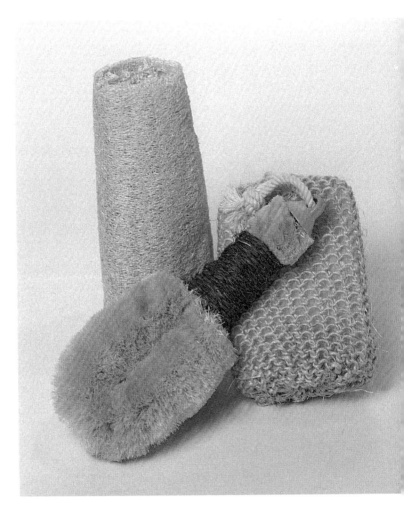

Start by filling a sink with hot herbal tea (see the Garden Medicine Cabinet, page 40)—enough to thoroughly soak an old sheet. (Because of the heat, you may need to wear rubber gloves to get your hands in there.) Wring out the tea and wrap the hot sheet around your body mummy-style, leaving head and arms out. Wrap a length of plastic wrap around the sheet. Lie down on a towel, and wrap it around you as well.

Lie back and relax with a cool compress on your forehead, taking sips of cold water. After 20 minutes (set an egg timer if you think you might fall asleep), unfurl your layers and follow up with a warm shower.

Mud

One of the newest trends in spa therapies is really among the oldest. As early as 120 B.C., the Romans mined the curative powers of mud from glacial lake beds. Renaissance physicians praised its healing properties, and today it still does wonders for rheumatism and a number of skin conditions such as eczema. Buttering nutrient-rich mud all over your body, or sinking into a tub full of primordial ooze does two things: first, the hot temperature gets you sweating and softens your pores; then the

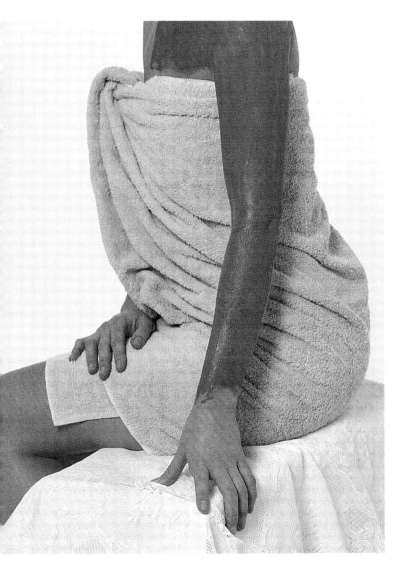

A body mask of warm mud softens pores and absorbs excess oil.

centuries-old organic matter draws out moisture and toxins as it dries. For that reason, mud is particularly good at absorbing oils from greasy skin. However, you can use mud as a hydrating mask by keeping the goop goopy. Preventing it from drying seals the moisture in.

Mud used in spa treatments, which geologically speaking is actually clay, is chock-full of plant extracts, inorganic substances such as salicylic acid, organic substances such as pectin, tannin and cellulose, as well as trace elements of silver, copper, gold and a number of vitamins. Clay is the product of thousands of years of erosion—ultra-fine rock particles that settle in layers. This molecular structure allows the clay-based mud to absorb your skin's water, oil and any impurities therein like a sponge.

Sitting in a mud bath is the ultimate in relaxation—it's a rare opportunity to lounge without aggravating any pressure points. More common are mud facials or body masks, where the mud is slathered all over your body, left to dry, then blasted off with a high-powered hose. At home you can try a number of mud products gleaned from mud supplies all over the world, including Jordan's legendary Dead Sea and a natural spa in Tuscany.

You can find mud facials in cosmetic sections of drug and department stores, fine salons and some health food stores. (Follow manufacturers' instructions.) But don't try your garden-variety dirt. Studies have shown that some mud can breed infection or, at the very least, skin irritation.

Thalassotherapy

Thalassotherapy—literally, "sea" therapy—uses the nutrients in sea water, seaweed and anything found in the sea to draw out toxins and cleanse the body. Seaweed wraps, saltwater sprays or sea-salt exfoliations are all thalassotherapy. Some cosmetics are made with seaweed, algae and kelp, but thalassotherapy is much more than a mere seaweed mask.

Originating in France at the turn of the last century, the first thalassotherapy treatment was a thermal salt bath. It was touted as a cure to whatever ailed you—rheumatism, gout, back and joint pain, circulatory problems and skin disorders. Today's true believers still regard thalassotherapy as an incredible cure-all, helping broken bones heal faster and even helping people quit smoking.

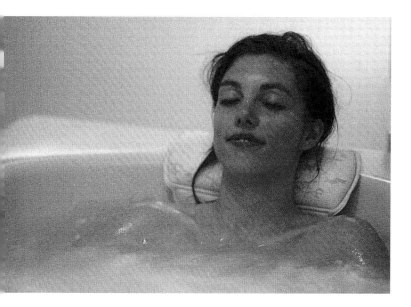

Thalassotherapy is part of the physician's standard arsenal in many European countries. Sea water is pumped directly to thalassotherapy clinics and used for baths and showers, among other treatments.

Though it's classified as an alternative therapy in North America, thalassotherapy remains a legitimate medical treatment in France to this day. Doctors are on-site at bona fide thalassotherapy centers, which pump water directly from the sea for their myriad treatments. Emphasis is on long-term therapy, not just short-term relief. As few as two sessions a year can reduce the need for anti-inflammatory drugs prescribed for arthritis, for example.

Therapy includes underwater massage, algae and mud body wraps, and aquafitness exercises performed in a saltwater pool. And whatever physiological effects the power of the sea may have, you can't argue with the stress-busting action. Lying in a tub of warm, pulsing water makes just about anyone relax.

The theory of thalassotherapy's potency makes sense—sea water has practically the same chemical make-up as human plasma, so the body easily absorbs the water, rich with nutrients from indigenous plants or matter. Sea water is loaded with all the minerals and trace elements that flow from the rivers to the sea. And because the body absorbs them through osmosis during a treatment, thalassotherapy is much more efficient than a vitamin or mineral supplement. The delicate mineral balance is the main reason water temperature is so crucial. The sea water must be at least 93°F for optimal skin penetration, but no hotter than 104°F or the beneficial organisms perish.

Hair Basics

Just like skin, the state of your hair plays an important role in conveying a good first impression. Healthy hair is also inextricably linked to a balanced diet and stress control. Those oil-producing sebaceous glands are attached to the hair follicles, so if stress causes you to break out, chances are it leads to greasy hair, too. People prone to dry skin may also fall prey to the ubiquitous dandruff, caused when red, flaky patches develop on the scalp and turn into a snowfall on your shoulders.

Hair is constantly growing, and even the healthiest head needs a regular trim to rejuvenate tired ends. Severe split ends, characterized by flyaway frizz, are caused by styling, brushing, rubbing hair dry and untangling knots. Blow-drying alone does not cause split ends; however, it can dry out the scalp and the heat can weaken the hair. Although too much brushing (more than your nightly 100 strokes) can lead to split ends, regularly running a brush through your hair distributes sebum along the hair shaft. It's your body's built-in hair conditioner.

Most people wash their hair too often. Exposing hair every day to even the mildest shampoo strips the hair of its natural oils, triggering the sebaceous glands to pump out more sebum. Conditioners don't actually "feed" hair in the way some manufacturers imply. Instead, the creams, which are often silicone-based, simply smooth over the cuticle scales on the surface of the hair. The result is shinier, sometimes stronger hair.

Hair Masks

It's easy to try to cover up bad hair. Take a hat or scarf, or any one of scads of hair products from sculpting mousses to freezing sprays. But fancy shampoos, conditioners and hair dressings are expensive. Before you shell out the big bucks, we have some intriguing low-tech solutions.

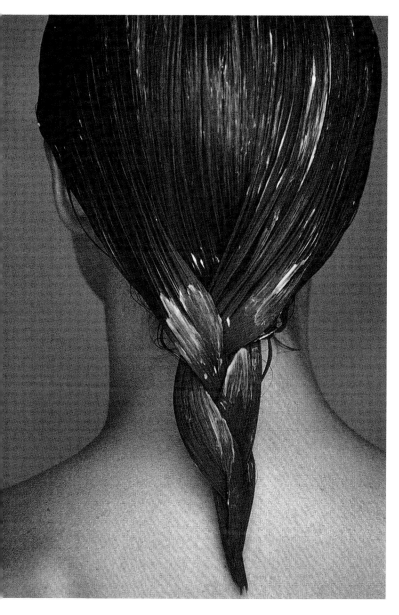

Hair masks help rejuvenate tired follicles and are usually best accompanied by a soothing scalp massage.

Masks aren't just good for your skin, they're also an excellent way to condition and revitalize hair. But don't merely slap the hair mask on. Just as the face is often ignored during massages, so too is the scalp. Head massages, as every good hairdresser knows, can relieve tension-induced headaches and help you relax. Use your fingers to work the mask into every square inch on your scalp.

FOR DRY HAIR

- Mix an avocado, an egg white and two generous tablespoons of baby oil in a blender. Apply on wet or dry hair, then wrap your head in plastic wrap for about 20 minutes. Sit in the sun or under a heat cap, then wash it out with warm water. Shampoo and condition.
- Mash a well-ripened banana with an equal part of tofu and apply to shampooed hair. The rich proteins help strengthen and moisturize weak hair. Slip on a bathing cap or plastic bag and step into a steamy shower, running the hot water over your head for about 20 minutes. Rinse well.

FOR OILY HAIR

If your hair tends toward the oily side, there are a couple of tacks you can take. First, how often do you wash your hair? Shampooing every day can cause your scalp's sebaceous glands to overcompensate for hair that's been stripped of its natural oils. Try gradually weaning yourself from a daily shampoo. If you have chronic bed-head, you can style your hair by misting with a spray bottle, or even better, switch to satin pillow cases. (They allow your hair to slide over the pillow, thus keeping its shape an extra day or two.) If that solution doesn't suit you, you can try the old lemon juice standard. On wet hair, work about a tablespoon of lemon juice into the roots. Let stand for about five minutes, then rinse. Your hair will be squeaky clean.

Soothing Scalp Massage

- Sitting in a comfortable chair, gently massage scalp for 15 minutes.
- Knead scalp with fingertips spread apart and stationary, working from front to back, following the path of circulation.
- For an invigorating treatment, apply lavender-sage oil and massage into hair with special emphasis on the ends.
- Cover head for 10 to 15 minutes with a shower cap, then shampoo.

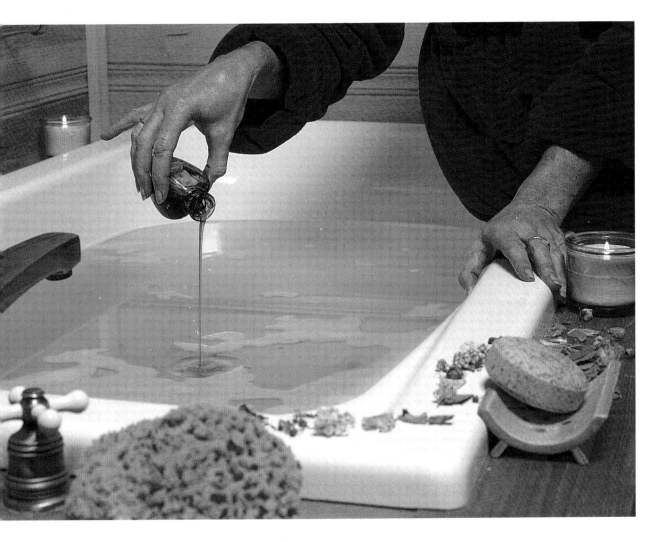

Aromatherapy

With alternative medical therapies gaining more and more accep-
tance today, it's no surprise aromatherapy is leading the way. To this
day, plants' pharmaceutical properties are being exploited to combat
everything from colds to cancer. Since Hippocrates, healers have
extracted essential oils from plant roots, wood, leaves, flowers or
fruit, and used them to cleanse and heal both body and mind, release
tension and even strengthen the immune system.

*A tablespoon of essential oil added to a
warm tub can turn your bathroom into
a spa.*

*Clary sage helps relieve insomnia and
headaches.*

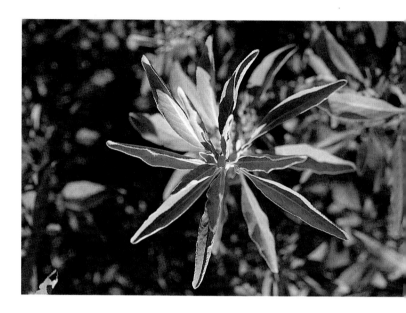

Many common medicines today use aromatherapy scents without knowing it. For instance, Vick's VapoRub's trademark
chest-opening scent is primarily eucalyptus, which is an age-old remedy for colds and flu. Most hot-drink cold remedies are flavored with
lemon, which is also a proven cold and flu fighter. Is it surprising
that lavender is used to fight depression? Doesn't a whiff of the heady
fragrance at once encourage you to breathe deeply and put a smile on
your face? But the scents are just an added bonus of aromatherapy—
it's the essential oils that do the work.

Because these aromatic oils are so concentrated, they are rarely
used on their own. Instead, a few drops of the essential oil are added
to a "carrier" oil, such as rapeseed, apricot kernel, jojoba, sweet
almond or even olive oil. This mixture is excellent for massage,
reflexology or shiatsu. Or a few drops can be diluted in your bath
water to make your evening soak more memorable.

Essential Oils and What They Do

Aromatherapy advocates say the fragrances released in these essential
oils treat more than 40 common health problems. Here's a list of
some of the most versatile oils and the complaints they are said to
help alleviate.

- Bergamot—Antiseptic, astringent, antidepressant. The characteristic fragrance of Earl Grey tea. Helps control acne and greasy hair.
- Black pepper—Relieves colds and flu, rheumatic pain and nausea.
- Cajeput—Excellent for rheumatism and arthritis.
- Caraway—Relieves and prevents nausea.
- Cedarwood—Intense scent penetrates nasal passages, relieving colds and flu.
- Chamomile—Antidepressant, but also soothes nerves. Good for relieving insomnia, headaches, rheumatism and arthritis, and PMS.
- Clary sage—Astringent, rejuvenating. Relieves insomnia, headaches, rheumatism and arthritis, and PMS.
- Cypress—Relieves insomnia and pain caused by varicose veins, and slows down cellulite development.
- Eucalyptus—Antiseptic and stimulating. Ideal for revitalizing sore muscles, treating headaches, colds and flu, rheumatism and arthritis.
- Frankincense—Excellent for colds and dry skin.
- Geranium—Astringent, diuretic, antidepressant. Also relieves colds and flu, rheumatism and arthritis, and PMS and helps slow down cellulite formation.
- Ginger—Relieves rheumatism and arthritis pain, as well as nausea.
- Jasmine—Antidepressant, aphrodisiac. Also stimulates uterine contractions.
- Juniper berry—Good for mental fatigue, insomnia, high blood pressure.
- Lavender—Antiseptic, analgesic. This is the wonder drug of aromatherapy. Calming lavender treats everything from insect bites to nausea, including headaches and PMS.
- Lemon—High Vitamin C makes it ideal for colds and flu. Also treats high blood pressure, varicose veins and rheumatism/arthritic pain.
- Mandarin—Good for high blood pressure and nausea.

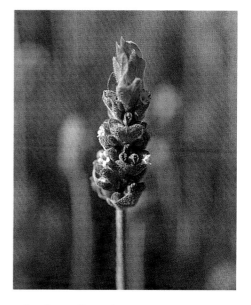

A few drops of lavender on your pillow helps cure insomnia.

- Marjoram—Analgesic, sedative. Lowers high blood pressure, relieves menstrual cramps and insomnia.
- Melissa (true)—Ideal for nausea and PMS.
- Neroli (orange blossom)—Sedative, aphrodisiac. Calms nerves and relieves insomnia.
- Peppermint—Antispasmodic, soothes and aids digestion. Also used for colds and flu.
- Rosemary—Stimulating, memory-booster. Alleviates rheumatism and arthritis, as well as varicose veins and cellulite production.
- Rose otto—Relieves depression, insomnia, nausea and PMS.
- Sandalwood—Invigorating, soothing scent treats depression, insomnia, nausea and PMS.
- Tea tree—Strongly medicinal oil ideal for colds and flu.
- Ylang-ylang—Treats depression, insomnia and high blood pressure.

Aromatherapy in Action

The potent, concentrated scents can be mixed with another oil, called a carrier oil, and used as a massage oil, or the undiluted scent can be added to the bath or used as an inhalation for the desired effect. Even a few drops in a dish of potpourri alter the room's atmosphere. Here are some ideas on how to benefit from aromatherapy every day.

WAKE-UP CALL Fill a spritzer with mineral water and add two teaspoons of clary sage oil. Spray face after cleansing.

RELAXING SOAK Add five drops each of lavender, clary sage, marjoram and chamomile oils to running bath water. Float the petals from three roses in the tub.

APHRODISIAC RUBDOWN A different kind of foreplay—add three drops of jasmine oil, twelve drops of sandalwood, twelve drops of ylang-ylang to mineral oil base; shake up, then knead mixture into your back and shoulders. Better yet, get that special someone to do it for you!

BRAIN BOOSTER Combine pure pine and peppermint oils in a small bottle; rub on temples, wrists and other pulse points to jump-start thinking. (Avoid eyes.)

PMS RELIEVER Add eight to ten drops of clary sage oil to warm water and soak a compress, then place on abdomen to relieve cramps.

DECONGESTANT Add a few drops of eucalyptus oil to a bowl of boiling water and drape a cloth over your head while breathing deeply.

AGING OR DRY SKIN TONIC Blend frankincense with Vitamin E and apricot kernel oil to rehydrate dry skin.

REVITALIZING SOAK Add eight to ten drops of geranium oil to the bath water for an anti-stress bath.

END INSOMNIA Sprinkle a few drops of lavender oil on your pillow for a better night's sleep.

SOOTHING SOAK Add just two drops of peppermint oil to the bath water for a cooling pick-me-up. (Avoid face.)

HAIR PICK-ME-UP Revitalize hair by rubbing rosemary oil into a wooden comb and use every day.

LOVE POTION Blend a drop of rose oil with jojoba oil and daub on the wrists and over the heart to ease grief or heartbreak.

INSTANT LOZENGE Rub tea tree oil on throat externally to relieve sore throat.

MENTAL RELIEF Put a drop of ylang-ylang in a teaspoon of carrier oil and apply to wrists to quell anger.

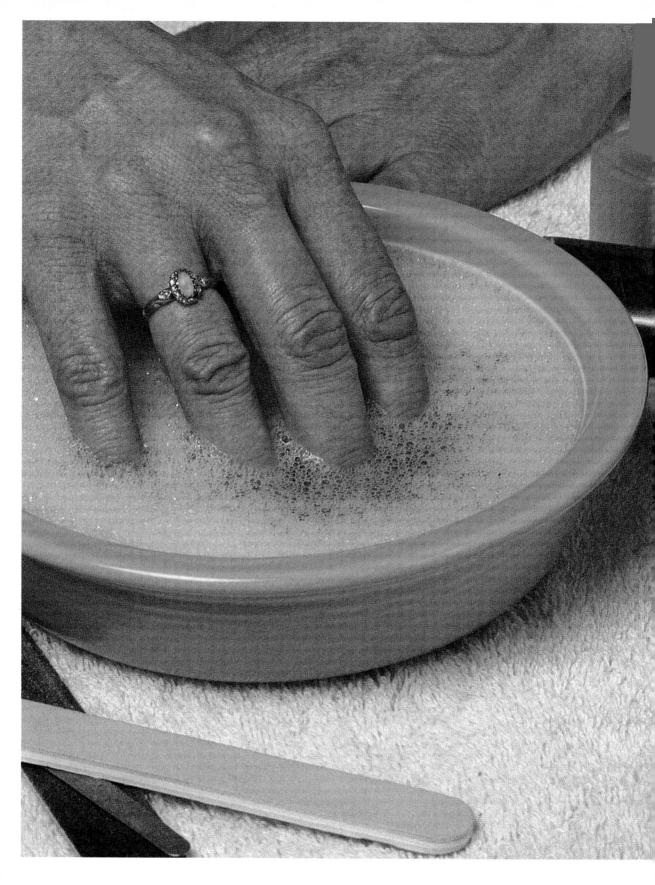

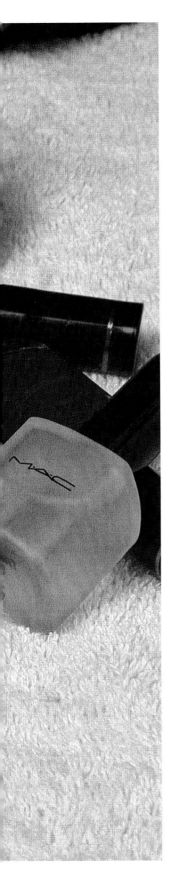

The Home Spa

9:00 a.m.	Breakfast
10:00 a.m.	Exercise
11:00 a.m.	Body Scrub and Shower
12:00 noon	Lunch
1:00 p.m.	Massage
3:00 p.m.	Manicure and Pedicure
4:00 p.m.	Facial, Scalp Treatment, Aromatherapy Tub

Furnish your bathroom with these spa essentials.

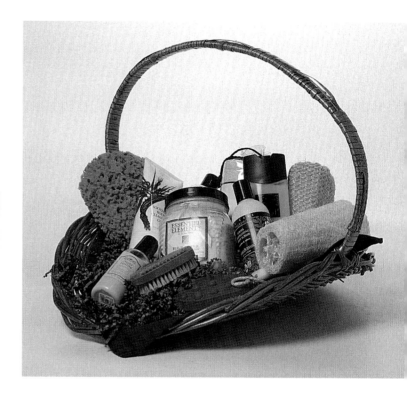

Block off a whole day to rejuvenate or just an hour for the treatment of your choice. We've outlined a typical spa-day program to make it easy for you. The tricky part is arranging to take the time off, be it from work or family, or both. Once you've read our simple but sumptuous recipes for destressing, we're sure you'll make the time.

Some tips on getting started:

- Fill a large pitcher with water and ice. Add a few lemon and cucumber slices, or blueberries and sliced strawberries if in season. Try to drink about eight glasses of water during the day to cleanse the toxins from your system. Water aids digestion and kidney function, hydrates muscles before, during and after exercise, and keeps skin healthier, too. If you find it hard to drink the recommended amount of water, you can supplement with fruits and vegetables, which are high in moisture content.
- Select some soothing music to play during the day. New-age instrumental collections are particularly effective, but choose whatever works for you.

- Set aside some long-forgotten reading material you've been meaning to get to (as long as it's not work-related). You can catch up during breakfast or lunch, or even during your tub at the end of the day.
- Buy some scented candles and potpourri to change the ambience. Candlelight in a darkened bathroom ensures a relaxing atmosphere.
- Indulge a little. A spa day should be unique, so why not cap it off with a chocolate truffle or a glass of champagne?
- Don't make any plans to go out that evening. Instead, let your body sink into sleep.

9:00 a.m. Breakfast

The most important meal of the day often gets short shrift in today's busy world of car pools, daycare and morning meetings. While business meetings used to be the preserve of lunch, the hastening work pace demands more hours in the day. Thus, the power breakfast meeting was born. For some, it just means an excuse to not eat breakfast; for others, it's a chance to finally start the day off with something other than black coffee.

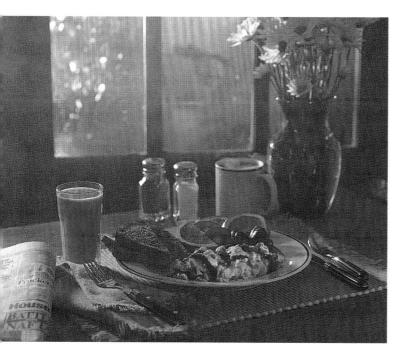

Start the day off with a balanced breakfast to provide energy and prevent overeating at lunch.

Adult metabolisms are a funny thing. Many people claim to be able to get by without breakfast, and when they do try to eat, they don't feel as sharp as they're used to feeling. We're not saying belly up to the breakfast bar for eight buttermilk pancakes. But you should recognize that even a piece of fruit with your coffee will help give you energy for the morning. That could help prevent overeating at lunch. If you're a calorie-counter, you should know that it's better to distribute calories throughout the day when your body is better able to burn them off—saving them up for a big dinner could result in an overall weight gain.

We've allotted an hour for breakfast to allow for preparation, cleanup and a relaxing pace. Take your time to enjoy the food. Set the table. Use the good silver and linen napkins. Prepare your favorite breakfast, or if you're in the mood to try something different, here are some suggestions:

Do you eat breakfast every day? People who eat breakfast tend to live longer than those who ignore early-morning nourishment.

—Sheila Cluff, The Oaks and
The Palms, California

Cereal with Milk Shake

1 frozen banana, broken into four or five pieces
1 cup skim milk
1 teaspoon vanilla extract

In blender, combine frozen banana with skim milk and vanilla. Pour over your favorite unsweetened cereal as an alternative to milk. For variety, try different frozen fruit, such as strawberries or peaches, or use fruit juice instead of milk.

Hot Cereal

¼ cup oatmeal
¼ cup oat bran
¼ cup skim milk   2 tablespoons ricotta cheese
1 tablespoon wheat germ   ½ teaspoon cinnamon
1 tablespoon wheat bran   ½ teaspoon pumpkin pie spice
                                            honey to taste

Cook oatmeal and oat bran with milk. Add wheat germ and wheat bran to the cooked cereal. Mix in ricotta cheese, cinnamon and pumpkin pie spice. Add honey to taste. For some crunch, add granola.

Low-fat Cheese Danish

whole-wheat pita

¼ cup cottage cheese

1 tablespoon raisins or chopped dates

1 teaspoon cinnamon

Slice pita in half and toast pockets in toaster. While toasting, mix remaining ingredients. Fill slightly toasted pita with mixture. Heat in microwave for 30 seconds, or under broiler for 2 minutes or until slightly browned and cheese is softened.

Breakfast Tips

- Fry an egg using non-stick spray instead of butter.
- Slice an orange for a healthy garnish. Combining iron-rich foods, such as whole grain breads or cereals, with Vitamin C helps your body better absorb the iron.
- Squeeze a little lemon juice over fruit salad to keep fruit from browning.
- Add dry cereal to yogurt for a change of texture.
- Ham is a leaner alternative to bacon.

10:00 a.m. Exercise

Get the blood flowing and break into a sweat with the exercise of your choice: a brisk one-hour walk; a light aerobic or weights work-out; a swim; ice skating.

11:00 a.m. Body Scrub and Shower

Exfoliate and cool down with one of our body treatments and a soothing shower.

You don't have to nibble on greens alone for your spa day lunch. Choose your menu wisely and you won't have to sacrifice flavor for fewer calories.

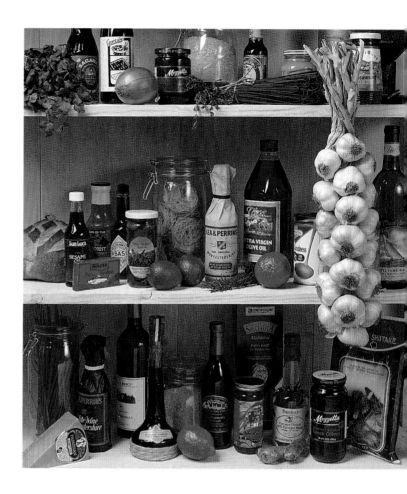

12:00 noon Lunch

The best part about going to a spa is having a license to wear a robe all day long. There's something utterly decadent in not getting dressed, and your home spa day should be no different. After your rejuvenating body scrub and shower you may feel like a nap—by all means, doze off if you do—but a little morsel of nourishment will help get you through your afternoon of massages and beauty treatments.

Healthy menus and nutritional counseling are basic features of most spas. We're not going to count calories (for some people, that's the cause of their stress!), but we are going to suggest a few menu ideas.

Menu Ideas

- Bed of mixed greens topped with broiled or grilled chicken breast and raspberry vinaigrette dressing.
- Omelette with red and green peppers.
- Toasted whole-grain bagel with low-fat cream cheese and sliced tomato.
- Sliced raw vegetables, plain or with low-fat dip.

For a drink, try your favorite fruit juice mixed with carbonated water or diet ginger ale. Equal parts orange juice, cranberry juice and your fizz of choice make a refreshing cocktail.

1:00 p.m. Massage

When following our massage instructions in Chapter 5, keep these tips in mind:

- Use a lubricant to help build up heat. You can buy a massage oil, or just use olive or almond oil mixed with an aromatherapy scent. (For more about aromatherapy oils, turn to page 92.) Avoid baby oil or any other petroleum-based products—they tend to evaporate more quickly and dry the skin.
- Take off all rings, watches and bracelets to avoid scratching yourself or your partner. As the massagee, don't forget to remove necklaces and earrings. Trim fingernails down to a workable length.
- Stick to massaging the soft tissue (muscle, skin, ligaments and tendons) and stay away from bone.
- Don't overwork your fingers. Instead, use your palms and the weight of your body to get more pressure.
- You can expect some pain in a massage, but if it becomes unbearable, say so and ask the massager to move on to another part of your body.
- A good massage will wake up muscles you forgot you had. It's normal to be a little tender for a day or two. If the soreness persists beyond a few days, see your doctor (or if the massage was from a professional, you might consider seeing him or her first).

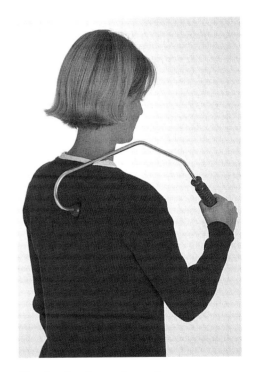

If you're planning a solo spa day, you may want to find a commercial massager for those hard-to-reach places.

- If you find a knot: A muscle knot forms when the tension has become so hard in a certain spot that the muscle tightens up, sometimes preventing you from moving freely. Finding one will undoubtedly make your partner wince, but working out a knot can produce a kind of enjoyable pain. Apply gentle pressure with your thumb, gradually increasing pressure until you feel the knot loosening. To apply more pressure, try using your elbow or your entire forearm.

3:00 p.m. Pedicure and Manicure

(Do the pedicure before the manicure to avoid ruining fingernail polish.)

Pedicure

In many European countries, a regular trip to the foot doctor is part of the health-care routine. The whole family gets nails trimmed, cuticles pushed down and stubborn calluses filed with a pumice stone. Keeping the nails trimmed helps shoes to fit properly, preventing possible bunion development. Neglecting calluses can sometimes result in corns, which have to be trimmed down or treated with medicated corn pads.

Everyone should have a professional pedicure at some time in his or her life. You can't beat the lower calf and foot massage, and let's face it, if you've been neglecting your feet all your life, you just might have to pay someone to touch them.

If you're on your own, or with a friend, start by soaking your feet in a tub of warm water laced with eucalyptus. Gehwol, a German line of foot-care products (translated, it means "walk well") is also good. After about 10 minutes of soaking, lift one foot onto your lap (or your friend's lap, if you are so lucky). With a pumice stone or foot file, start rubbing away at the calluses on your heel and ball of the foot. A professional may use a straight razor to shave away slivers of dead skin, but don't try this at home. Then use a cuticle cream to soften the cuticles; a Vitamin E capsule will also do the job. With an orange stick, gently push the cuticles down, never cutting them. File nails, clipping any ornery, extra-long ones. Finish the job with a

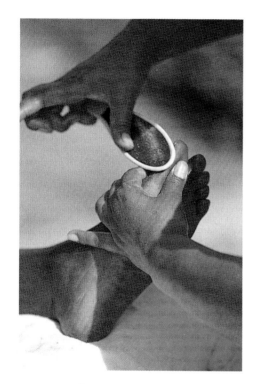

Even if you're not into painting your toenails, you should pay attention to those thick, hard calluses. Soak your feet in warm, soapy water to soften them, then gently rub with a pumice stone or file, as seen here.

liberal application of moisturizer or, for really dry skin, vegetable or olive oil. Peppermint-scented foot cream or oil is especially invigorating. Then stuff your feet into a pair of thick, absorbent socks to retain the moisture. Wear them as long as you can, ideally overnight, for soft and tender tootsies. (If you wish to paint your toenails, do it after filing and clipping them, then let polish dry—about 15 minutes—before continuing with moisturizer and socks.)

Manicure

Not everyone is into flirty red nail polish, but a manicure is more than 10 daubs of color. In fact, the North American custom of shaking hands upon meeting someone demands that we at least keep nails trim and clean. (The Europeans' cheek-kissing lets them off easy.) Occupational hazards of washing dishes and working at a computer keyboard, to name two examples, often bear themselves out with soft hangnails or brittle split nails.

The cuticle's job is to protect the nail from bacteria. Letting them get overgrown, however, can lead to hardening; then you're left with those painful and red puffy nail beds.

A manicure is most successful when someone else is doing it—being able to alternate from hand to hand allows for better timing. Besides, while a manicure should be part of your regular grooming, it should also give your hands a rest.

CUTICLES: After removing any existing nail polish with rubbing alcohol or a commercial nail polish remover, soak your hands in hot soapy water to soften the cuticles. After about 10 minutes, take one hand and rub additional cuticle softener into the nail beds. With an orange stick, push down cuticles, trimming any hard ends that may catch on clothes or that might be tempting to pull off. Soaking the hands should also encourage dead skin on the fingertips to loosen. Carefully trim it off with nail scissors. Return hand to the warm water and repeat these steps on the other hand.

NAILS: Manicurists almost always use emery boards, not the metal files with the point at the end for cleaning under nails. File each fingernail, working in one direction only to prevent splitting. Some

Foot massagers like this, or even a simple tennis ball, can soothe sore spots on the souls of your feet.

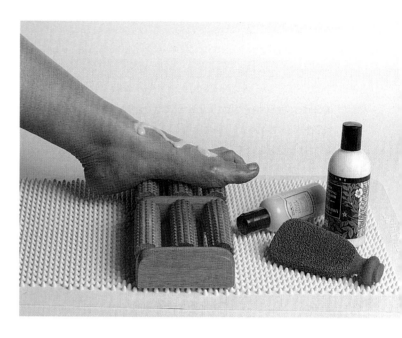

people like a squarer look, or you can follow the natural curve of the nail. Slide the file under and behind the nail, instead of flat against the top. This shapes the nail so that it is slightly thinner at the tip, which further prevents splitting. Using the orange stick again, gently remove any nail dust from under the nails. Return hand to the soapy water and repeat steps on other hand.

MOISTURIZE: Ah, the hand massage. Choose your favorite hand cream or moisturizer and apply generously, working it in to each knuckle and muscle.

BUFF AND POLISH: A clear base coat of polish is the least anyone should do to protect his or her nails from the elements. It also doesn't have to go on too cleanly, since it dries flat. Buff with a nail buffer to the desired shine.

A clear lacquer or polish, however, needs to be applied with a bit more care. Most manicurists leave about a hair's width unpolished on either side of the nail and at the cuticle. It makes the nail look longer and also allows for cuticle and nail growth.

Deluxe Hand/Foot Treatment

A hot paraffin wax treatment is an easy way to give new life to battered appendages.

First, melt paraffin wax (available at grocery stores) in a pot or disposable metal food container. Massage olive oil into clean hands or feet.

Dip hands or feet into the slightly cooled wax four to five times to give a strong coat. Cover them with a plastic bag and wrap with a towel if desired. While the paraffin cools and hardens into a waxy glove, relax for about 15 minutes.

Unwrap, then peel off the "glove." Hands or feet will be soft and sleek for approximately two weeks.

4:00 p.m. Facial, Scalp Treatment, Aromatherapy Tub

Finish off your spa day with a combination aromatherapy tub, facial and hair treatment. Start by lighting some fragrant candles and selecting some soothing music. Draw a bath of hot water (by the time you get in, it will be pleasantly warm, and the hot water will turn your bathroom into a mini-steamroom). Add a few drops of the aromatherapy scent of your choice—lavender or chamomile are especially soothing (see guide on page 92). You can also add a quarter cup of sea salts, European mineral salts or mineral-rich seaweed (algae) powder.

Apply your favorite moisturizer or face mask (try one of ours from Chapter 5), following the manufacturer's instructions, if it's store-bought. With a natural bristle bath brush, dry-brush your entire body using circular motions starting at your feet and working upwards to the chest. This stimulates circulation and the lymphatic system, which speeds up the body's internal cleansing.

For an inexpensive but effective hot oil hair conditioner, massage in a few tablespoons of body massage oil or olive oil on wet hair. Or try one of the hair masks in Chapter 5. Wrap your head in a hot towel to seal in moisture.

Always replace the moisture lost through exfoliating with a good moisturizer.

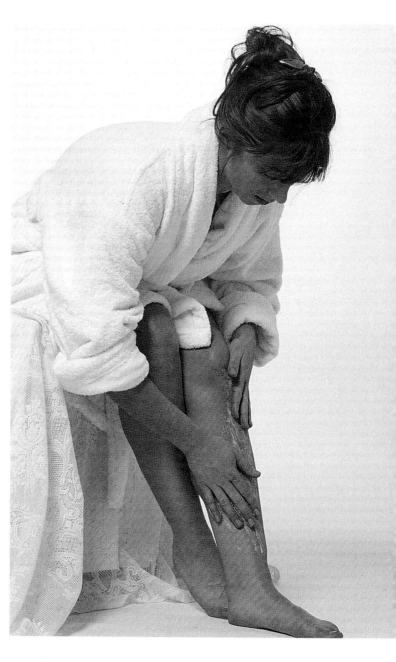

Fill a bowl with ice water and set it within arm's reach before you lower yourself into the tub. An inflatable bath pillow is a comfy accessory, but you can also slide a rolled-up towel under your neck (it will get wet). First immerse a face towel in the bath water, then wring it out. Lay the rolled, steaming towel around your face, leaving the mouth and nose clear for breathing. Then take four cotton make-up remover pads and soak them in the chilling water. Place two pads on each eye—one right on top, one towards the temple. The coolness helps take down any swelling or puffiness and also provides a stimulating contrast to the hot wrap. Relax in your tub for about 15 minutes, then slowly lift yourself out. Let the water out and have a warm shower to rinse off hair treatment and face mask.

Pat your body dry—don't rub—and finish off with one final application of moisturizer. Rest for at least another 15 minutes. In about an hour, your skin and soul will be smooth and marvelously mellow.

Where to Find It

Bath and Beauty Products

Aveda
The aromatherapy giant. All extracts from plants are organic.
800-283-3224

Bath & Body Works
Bath products created with ingredients from America's heartland.
800-395-1001

The Bayou Blending Company
Bath oils, pure aromatherapy oils, bath salts.
800-764-8361

The Body Shop
This international retailer of skin and hair care products has everything from aromatherapy treatments to bath and massage oils to invigorating facial masks.
800-541-2535

Essential Elements
Essential oils, bath salts, shower and bath gels.
800-908-4009

The Golden Door Products
Bath and body products inspired by a California orange grove.
800-231-1444

Green Valley Spa Products
Bath products created using ingredients from the Utah desert.
800-237-1068

Kerstin Florian Inc.
Mineral, herbal and aromatherapy bath products.
800-233-6629

Planet Emu
Real emu oil, which can be used for relief of sore muscles and joints, dry skin, fine lines and wrinkles, and other ailments.
800-373-4011

Renaissance Spa Treatments
"Bath of the Month Club" members get monthly bath and body products from spas around the world.
800-406-2284

Totally for Men
Shave creams, after-shave balms, and body wash and lotion created just for men.
800-820-7350

Mud Products

Aveda
Their Deep Cleansing Herbal Clay Masque takes only five minutes to cleanse and purify the skin.
800-283-3224

Bloom
A dark mud mask made from the thick, rich mud of Jordan's Dead Sea.
800-658-3708

Chattem
Their MUDD products are some of the most widely available and least expensive masks. Comes in three formulations.
800-745-2429

Ecco Bella Botanicals
Their Aromatherapy Glacial Mud contains aloe to counteract the drying effects of the mud.
201-696-7766

Glen Ivy
Three different clay masks for different skin types, as well as tanning products and bath salts.
800-454-8772, ext. 540

Kerstin Florian Inc.
A deep-cleaning Black Mud Masque made from ancient moor mud and full of minerals and trace elements.
800-233-6629

Louison Bobet
Their Super Fine Green Clay is pure kaolin that has been sun-dried to a fine powder.
719-538-1909

Moor-Life
Mud products made from the 2,000-year-old Neydhardting Moor of Austria. Baths, masks and soaps contain over 700 herbs and plants.
800-666-7987

Terme di Saturna
The Purifying Thermal Facial Mud comes from the banks of a 3,000-year-old natural spa in Tuscany famed for its thermal waters.
800-386-3021

Seaweed Products

Bain de Terre
Their Marine Botanicals line incorporates kelp and sea extracts to soothe and moisturize the skin.
800-242-9283

Bare Escentuals
A full line of seaweed products that includes bubble bath, shower gel and a chunky loofah soap.
800-227-3990

The Body Shop
A newly introduced line of seaweed products, called Marinis, includes oils, soaps and shower gels.
800-541-2535

Louison Bobet
This French company offers a line of four seaweed products designed to combat cellulite.
713-538-1909

Phytomer
Sea-based bath products made from seaweed, seawater and blue algae.
800-227-8051

Repêchage Day Spa
This New York City spa carries a whole line of seaweed and sea water body and facial treatments.
800-284-5044

Thalgo
Their rich Thalassobath is one of the truest home thalassotherapy treatments.
800-228-4254

Accessories

Aquassage, Inc.
Non-slip rubber mats with nodules that massage your feet while you shower.
503-968-2143

Crystal Candles
Long-lasting candles (up to 50 hours each) scented with fragrance from essential oils.
602-569-0090

Earth Solutions
Their Scentball plugs into any outlet and diffuses the scent of your favorite essential oil by heating it on a cotton pad. They also make Carscenter, which plugs into your car's cigarette lighter.
800-555-1174

The Herb Farm
Maker of Sleep Bunny, a must-have for insomniacs. This soft toy is filled with aromatic, calming herbs such as lavender and hops to help you get to sleep.
800-866-4372

Lanaform
European sandals are designed to stretch and tone little-used muscles along the back of the calf, thigh, hip and rear.
800-309-9872

Susan Dunn Spawear
Offers cotton-and-terry robes, slippers and other wraps for a real spa experience at home.
800-772-2772

Tender Loving Things
Creator of the Hit the Spot! self-massager, which helps loosen tight muscles in the shoulders and back.
800-486-2896

Twirly Towel
This handy, elasticized hair towel is secured with a button so you can take a bath or give yourself a facial without fear of it sliding off.
800-527-8430

Variel Health International
Makers of the aromaSpa steam capsule, a telephone-booth-sized chamber that acts as your own private sauna.
800-892-7662

Workout Equipment

Free Weights and Weight Machines
Hoist Fitness Systems
800-548-5438

Ivanko Barbell Co.
800-247-9044

Pacific Fitness
800-722-3482

Parabody
800-328-9714

Paramount Fitness Equipment
800-421-6242

Perfect Flex 2000
800-997-3999

Tuff Stuff
800-824-5210

Vectra Fitness Inc.
800-283-2872

Cardio Equipment
Aerobics Inc.
201-256-5391

Bodyguard Fitness
800-944-3144

Diamondback
805-484-4450

Landice Inc.
201-927-9010

Life Fitness
800-735-3867

NordicTrack
800-892-2174

Precor
206-486-9292

Schwinn
303-939-0100

Spirit
800-258-4555

StairMaster
800-782-4799

Tectrix Fitness Equipment
800-767-8082

Trotter
800-677-6544

True Fitness Technology
800-426-6570

Tunturi Inc.
800-827-8717

Unisen Inc.
800-228-6635

Versa Climber
800-237-2271

Accessories
Bollinger
Maker of thickly padded, vinyl
aerobic floor mats.
800-527-1166

Collage Video
Their catalogue, *The Complete Guide
to Exercise Videos*, offers hundreds of
tapes covering all facets of exercise.
800-433-6769

ExerWise Productions
Distributors of Irwin Schwartz's
excellent video *At Home with Your
Weight Training Machine.*
800-732-6317

SPRI
Manufacturers of so-called resistance
bands, which promote muscle toning.
800-222-7774

Theraband
Like SPRI, Theraband also makes
elastic tubing for strength workouts.
800-321-2135

Clothing
Danskin
800-288-6749

Reebok
800-454-4005